MW00444702

A PERFECTLY STRIKING DEPARTURE

A PERFECTLY STRIKING DEPARTURE

*Surgeons and Surgery at the
Peter Bent Brigham Hospital
1912–1980*

Nicholas L. Tilney, M.D.

Science History Publications/USA
Sagamore Beach
2006

First published in the United States of America
by Science History Publications/USA
a division of Watson Publishing International
Post Office Box 1240, Sagamore Beach, MA 02562-1240, USA
www.shpusa.com

Library of Congress Cataloging-in-Publication Data

Tilney, Nicholas L.
    A perfectly striking departure : surgeons and surgery at the
  Peter Bent Brigham Hospital, 1912–1980 / Nicholas L. Tilney.
      p. cm.
    Includes bibliographical references (p.   ).
    ISBN 0-88135-382-5 (alk. paper)
    1. Peter Bent Brigham Hospital. Dept. of Surgery—History.   I. Title.

RD28.A1T55 2006
617.092'274461—dc22

                         2006045026

Designed and typeset by Publishers' Design and Production Services, Inc.
Manufactured in the USA.

*Dedicated to the surgeons
of today and tomorrow . . .*

CONTENTS

"It is often said or implied that in our profession, a man cannot be practical and scientific; science and practice seem to people to be incompatible. Each man, they say, must devote himself to the one or the other. The like of this has long been said, and it is sheer nonsense."

Sir James Paget, 1896

"The purest experiment in treatment may still be conscientious; my business is to take care of life, and to do the best I can think of for it. Science is properly more scrupulous than dogma. Dogma gives a charter to mistake. But the very breadth of science is a contest with mistakes, and must keep the conscience alive."

George Eliot, *Middlemarch*

PREFACE

THE PETER BENT BRIGHAM HOSPITAL, the newly built teaching arm of the Harvard Medical School, received its first patient in 1913. It merged into a larger institution, the Brigham and Women's, in 1980. During the seven decades of its existence the ongoing contributions of the faculty in the Department of Surgery represented, in microcosm, the development of the entire field. Operative procedures increased in scope and sophistication commensurate with more comprehensive diagnosis and care of abnormalities that involved all bodily organs and systems. Clinician-scientists introduced the new subject of neurosurgery, designed operations to treat both congenital and acquired heart disease, characterized body composition, and calculated the dynamics of fluids and salts during injury and convalescence. With increasing success, they replaced non-functioning organs with the healthy organs of others. Anesthesia, patient safety, asepsis, effective blood replacement, intensive care, and accurate monitoring of the physiological changes of illness and convalescence improved. In parallel with these patient-based advances, unique and relevant bio-sciences emerged.

As the significance of these events to the field of surgery as a whole and the setting in which they occurred should not be forgotten, I have tried to portray the spirit and contributions of the Brigham Department of Surgery during its 70-year existence, a period in which new ideas, technologies, and applicable biologies supported and embellished each other in comprehensive, specialized, and increasingly effective care of the ill. My long clinical attachment to this particular university hospital and my investigative collaborations with talented scientists on the faculty of the adjacent medical school provided me with much background as I had heard about earlier events and improvements in surgery and surgical biology from my teachers and had experienced directly, or at least peripherally, novel concepts and realities that came into being during my career. It also has become increasingly clear that I, like many others of my professional generation and perhaps without realizing all of its ramifications, had lived through a period of growth and discovery so unique that it may never be repeated. It seems correct to record them.

This account is an amalgamation of pertinent publications, annual reports, research grants, and letters collected over many years. Equally as important are the reminiscences, memoires, interactions, and friendships with many of the principles who provided anecdotes, stories, and leads into finding long-buried information. It was a rewarding journey.

I wrote *The Fabric of the Body* both for the surgeons, physicians, investigators, patients, and friends familiar with the Brigham, and for a broader audience interested in the course of clinical surgery and its associated sciences that developed over the bulk of a remarkably productive century. In particular, I wrote it for our surgical successors who work in larger and more complex institutions under different circumstances and conditions than did their professional ancestors. These include younger colleagues, residents, and students who often assimilate only snippets of prior events, hear the gossip and folklore surrounding parts of the subject, gape at the eccentricities of the pioneers, and take for granted innovations and advances that have now become routine.

I am grateful to colleagues and friends who reviewed relevant parts of the developing manuscript and provided information regarding their own areas of expertise. I am particularly appreciative of the efforts of Robert Bartlett, Murray Brennan, the late Chilton Crane, Robert Demling, Philip Drinker, Joseph Garfield, Alfred Morgan, John Mannick, Curtis Prout, John Rowbotham, John Sanders, David Sugarbaker, and the late Carl Walter. David Brooks loaned me important letters to and from the first superintendent of the Brigham, his great grandfather. Tristam Dammin generously provided rare photographs. My teacher and mentor, Joseph Murray, has generously given support and encouragement to me for decades, while the enthusiasm and élan of the late Francis Moore firmly shaped my career as a surgical academic and made my professional life exceptionally enjoyable and challenging. John Mannick has been a constant source of advice. Michael Zinner, the current Surgeon-in-Chief of the Brigham and Women's Hospital, has kindly provided me time and space to produce this book. Brian Bator of the Photography Department at the Brigham has been of immeasurable aid in restoring old photos and providing new ones. The resources of the Countway Library of Medicine at Harvard Medical School are limitless. It is an unending pleasure to wander around its stacks and find the needed books and papers regardless of the years in which they were published. The Rare Book Department is a treasure trove of unpublished letters and memorabilia. My secretaries, Brenda Hayslett and Deb McLaughlin, had cheerfully transcribed drafts of chapters.

Several senior Brigham surgical faculty members provided generous financial support for this project. These include Peter Black of Neurosurgery, David Brooks of SOBSA, Elof Erikson of Plastic Surgery, Lawrence Cohn of Cardiac Surgery, Francis Moore, Jr. of General Surgery, and David Sugarbaker of Thoracic Surgery. I am most grateful to them.

The debt I owe my family is incalculable. My daughters, Rebecca, Louise, Victoria, and Frances, have put up with the exigencies of a surgical career and cheerfully supported and enhanced my academic efforts while pursuing their own varied lives and vocations. My gratitude to them is boundless. My wife, Mary, has not only created an atmosphere of personal calm and happiness, but as supervisor of the Surgical Research Laboratory at Harvard Medical School and manager of research grants over several decades, has made my own investigative efforts possible.

A PERFECTLY
STRIKING
DEPARTURE

CHAPTER 1

A VERY IMPORTANT STEP

IN HIS FIRST *Annual Report to the Board of Trustees* of the Peter Bent Brigham Hospital, Harvey Cushing, the recently named Surgeon-in-Chief and Moseley Professor of Surgery at Harvard Medical School, noted that Mary Agnes Turner, a 45-year-old woman from nearby Roxbury was the first patient to enter the still unfinished institution on January 22, 1913 for removal of large and symptomatic varicose veins.[1] The entire surgical staff participated. Cushing, a pioneer in neurosurgery recently recruited from Johns Hopkins, made the incision as a symbolic gesture. David Cheever performed the operation with the aid of Conrad Jacobson, a resident. Walter Boothby administered open drop ether. John Homans, the other general surgeon, gave advice. And despite this plethora of expertise, Mrs. Turner did well.

Two years later the professor was able to report that 2184 admissions had filled the 110 beds of the new institution.[2] While the numbers appear mundane at retrospective glance, many individuals both within and outside the Boston community had expended a good deal of time and effort to achieve them.

TO UNDERSTAND MORE COMPLETELY the hospital that Mrs. Turner entered for her surgery, it might be well to review briefly the dynamics behind its gestation and birth. The period leading up to the opening of the Brigham was one of reform in medicine and medical education in the United States. Much of the impetus had arisen in Baltimore. The Johns Hopkins Hospital and its medical school, financed by the seven million dollars left years before by its founder, was formed in 1886 and opened in 1893. Its president, Daniel Coit Gilman, one of the foremost educators in the country, appointed an enthusiastic and prescient coterie of four distinguished academic professors identified through national searches. Basing their improvements primarily on the

1

highly structured curriculum of German universities, they revamped completely the entrance requirements (a college degree would be necessary), designed a four-year course of study for the medical students, and instituted a pattern of residency training that related knowledge from the basic sciences directly to clinical questions. All-powerful, full-time professors were placed in charge of the departments and their faculties, in contrast to other American university hospitals that continued to adhere to the British-based system in which a handful of practitioners ran individual services or spent several months each year in private practice.

Other organizational changes were also evolving. Economic improvements reduced the bloated numbers of commercial institutions throughout the country, many of which sold diplomas through the mail. The Flexner Report of 1910, *Medical Education in the United States and Canada*, did much to alter the status quo from an uncontrolled proprietary system to one that was increasingly the responsibility of the universities. With more standardized training the profession became more cohesive. The plethora of patent medicines, so prevalent in earlier decades, came under state regulation. Numbers of specialists increased, charlatans and quacks declined. Infant mortality diminished, life expectancy lengthened. Public health measures began to control the spread of infectious diseases. Anesthesia and surgery improved. The American faith in simplicity and common sense began to yield to a celebration of science and technology. The prestige of the medical profession increased; to become a doctor was a desirable career.

Several factors stimulated the shift toward the modern teaching hospital. These included the obvious success of the Hopkins prototype in Baltimore, the findings of the Flexner Report, increasing emphasis on scientific investigations into the diagnosis and treatment of disease, and the interest of both students and faculty in improving care. Important partnerships and mergers were announced following the association between the Brigham and Harvard Medical School, most notably those between Columbia's medical school and Presbyterian Hospital in New York, and Washington University and Barnes Hospital in St. Louis. Additional models appeared. By the 1930s, American medical education had improved dramatically.[3]

With these changes providing a fresh force in American medicine, the time was propitious for the creation of a large academic medical complex in Boston. The Peter Bent Brigham and its predominantly

Hopkins-trained faculty refined the new concept substantially, blending organized residency training under a dedicated staff with comprehensive patient care through clinical observation, accurate laboratory determinations, biologic knowledge, and technical improvements. The two institutions, one in Baltimore and the other in Boston, in concert with others that gradually began to follow their lead, began to produce important and continuing advances in diagnosis and treatment, education, and investigation.

Considerations about a final location for a proposed teaching hospital for Harvard Medical School had been ongoing for several years. Founded in 1782, the school had already occupied several locales in Boston, across the Charles River and away from the main campus and the remainder of its graduate sections in Cambridge. A move in 1883 to yet another downtown location with appropriate panoply to celebrate its 100th anniversary caused much rejoicing among the professors and the students as "the considerably improved accommodation on Boylston St. was expected to be the home of medicine for generations."[4] Although professors and students remained at that site for 23 years, all soon realized that the "considerably improved accommodations" lacked both laboratory space and spare land for expansion. Even the curriculum was a source of controversy, with several of the less scientifically oriented faculty reproaching some of their more serious colleagues "for encouraging [their] students to fritter away their time in the labyrinths of chemistry and physiology.' " Despite the presence of several distinguished personalities on the faculty, the school was not flourishing.

Like most other comparable institutions in the United States, Harvard Medical School was essentially "a money making institution not much better than a diploma mill," sponsored by a few individuals of the Boston medical establishment of the time, their families, and their friends.[5] In addition, because the major hospitals already existing in Boston—the Massachusetts General Hospital (MGH) and the Boston City—insisted on autonomy for both their administrative and their staff appointments, the school was completely dependent upon their choices for its own faculty. Cronyism often resulted.

Not until Charles William Eliot, a mathematician and scientist at the Massachusetts Institute of Technology, became President of Harvard University in 1869 did the situation improve. Reacting against the established forces, Eliot instituted a series of far-reaching educational and financial reforms to raise the standards of this weak section of the university. Supported quickly thereafter by similar changes at the Universities of Pennsylvania and Michigan, these included strict entrance requirements, a more organized and stringent course structure, a comprehensive curriculum presented over a three-year period, and written examinations. While many of the faculty opposed such innovations, particularly a conservative faction from the MGH led by a particularly forceful surgeon, academic performance improved dramatically. The issue of who was to pick the professional personnel, however, remained problematic for some years.

In 1900, Eliot and his delegation received word of a plan to acquire a property large enough for an expanded medical school and an adjacent hospital nearby the already proposed private New England Baptist and New England Deaconess Hospitals. Of three possible locations, the most desirable included part of the Ebenezer Francis estate in Roxbury, a tract of land "overlooking the vast and liquid acres of old Back Bay and Muddy River." This was in the Longwood area of Boston, named after Napoleon Bonaparte's site of exile on St. Helena. It seemed a good choice. "Part of this district is close to the centre of the City's population and at the same time land values are comparatively low. It is convenient of access for both patients and doctors, and is in the general direction of the City's growth. In addition, neither the City Hospital nor the Massachusetts General Hospital are near to this section."[6] Potential competition was a consideration even then.

While a substantial endowment was already in place, considerably more money was needed to build and equip the intended Longwood complex. The prospect of an underfinanced multimillion project was frightening. Even Eliot became nervous. But the moment to raise funds was propitious as the nation prospered in an age of large enterprises initiated and guided by men of great wealth. The Boston philanthropist, Major Henry Lee Higginson, formed a syndicate of receptive colleagues who began to identify potential benefactors for the project. Plans were drawn. The style of the proposed buildings, massive and lacking elaborate detail, copied structures of ancient Greece. The laboratory doorways duplicated those discovered in Assos by the American Archeological Expedition 20 years before.

J. Pierpont Morgan, John D. Rockefeller, and Mrs. Collis P. Huntington of New York, plus several benefactors in Boston examined the plans. They all promised financial aid. The land was bought and the structures designed. "By most accounts, the first meeting between Morgan and the faculty members lasted only five minutes. Morgan strode into the office, looked at the architectural plans lying on the table, and said, 'Those are good-looking buildings. How much will the administration and the two adjoining buildings cost?' Without receiving a definite answer from his incredulous hosts, he added 'Send me your architects. Good morning, gentlemen.' "[7] Building began in 1903, using Italian marble discarded by the New York Public Library because it was the wrong color; it was acquired at a bargain price. The new facility was completed in 1906.

The prospect of a university hospital for the Harvard Medical School was increasingly attractive to those on its faculty who favored the Longwood venture and to their supporters on the Harvard Corporation. About that time and almost by happenstance, they became aware of the terms of Peter Bent Brigham's will, stipulating the founding of a hospital "dedicated to the care of sick persons in indigent circumstances in the county of Suffolk." With this potential carrot dangling before them, they opened discussions with the executors of

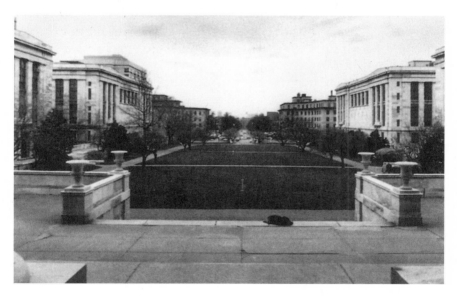

FIGURE 1.1   The new Harvard Medical School from the portico of the administration building.

his estate toward creating a teaching institution adjacent to the new school. Indeed, by 1910, just before the actual ground breaking took place, the original trust had grown to $5.3 million, almost one quarter of the total endowment of the university itself. As a further inducement to any skeptics on the board of trustees of the intended hospital, Harvard offered them both a portion of the land, and for the first time in its history, assigned unrestricted funds to the overall venture. This largess caused those who still doubted the possibilities to "begin to think seriously of a new physical plant some removed from Boylston Street only *after* they had reached an informal agreement with the executors of Mr. Brigham's will respecting a hospital which, from the Harvard point of view, would be a teaching as well as a charitable institution."[8]

Although the cautious "executors of Mr. Brigham's will" agreed to a close relationship with the medical school, they insisted on continuing independence for their institution. And at the same time disquiet arose in the corridors of power of the State House that care of the indigent might not only take place in a teaching hospital filled with trainees but that money designated for the benefit of the impoverished sick of the city might ultimately find its way into Harvard's coffers. This latter prospect was anathema to the politicians! The charge, such as it was, was led by a young alderman, James Michael Curley. Later becoming one of Boston's most famous (or infamous) mayors, he was once re-elected from jail.

The philosophic contest of wills between hospitals and medical schools was not unique to Harvard and its overtures to the potential Brigham Hospital. Although hospitals in the United States had cooperated in the education of future physicians since the Civil War, they had consciously limited their involvement with students, feeling that their primary responsibility was to their patients. The efforts of the educational institutions, in contrast, were dedicated to teaching and research.[9] Despite persistent overtures by medical schools throughout the country for more visibility on the clinical wards, patient-based teaching remained rudimentary during the early years of the twentieth century. The innovative Johns Hopkins was the only example of a university-owned hospital dedicated both to teaching and to care of the sick.

Interestingly, despite subsequent decades of productivity that combined the traditional academic tripartite credo of patient care, teaching, and research, this dichotomy in roles between hospital and medical school still exists, aggravated further in recent years, perhaps, by the financial and temporal demands and strategies of cost containment. Harvard, for instance, still has no University Hospital, but is served by several affiliated but autonomous institutions, each with its own board of trustees and administration.

NEGOTIATIONS BETWEEN THE UNIVERSITY corporation and the hospital trustees continued to move forward with Brigham's bequest as the cornerstone. Indeed, "historical evidence strongly supports the notion that the huge medical center would not likely have assumed its present form had not the will of a man born in Vermont provided for the creation of a great new hospital. As early as 1900, the Peter Bent Brigham Hospital—still 13 years short of existence—became the key factor in the overall complex design."[10] Reality began to overtake conjecture when the new buildings of the Harvard Medical School opened their doors and it became apparent that the proposed teaching hospital would arise across Shattuck Street a few years later, fully mature, heavily endowed, and able to attract a select staff of physicians and surgeons of national stature, free from the parochialism of the closed professional and social élite of the existing Boston medical establishment.

The man from Vermont after whom the hospital was named was born in 1807.[11] Peter Bent Brigham, one of the younger children of a family that had moved north from Massachusetts a decade before, spent his childhood in relative poverty with his widowed mother and eight siblings. Hoping to improve his expectations, he started for Boston by horseback at age 17, finally arriving in the city by foot and virtually penniless. Beginning by selling oysters and fish from a wheelbarrow, he eventually bought and operated a successful downtown restaurant. A shrewd investor, he ultimately became a millionaire in real estate and as director of a local railroad.

Within a few years, his nephew also left Vermont to begin work at his uncle's restaurant. A similar type of upright and community-spirited man, he eventually opened his own restaurant and hotel. Also making much money in local real estate, he set aside ample funds to start the Robert Breck Brigham Hospital in 1914 for those with arthritic disorders.[12] Three-quarters of a century later, these two neighboring institutions merged with a third to form the Brigham and Women's Hospital (BWH). This has become a commanding presence in the delivery of health care, particularly after its more recent affiliation with the powerful MGH in 1994.

DURING THE YEARS OF PLANNING for the proposed 110-bed teaching hospital, considerations about the heads of the proposed departments, medicine, surgery, pathology, and radiology, began to take administrative precedence. In surgery, glowing embers of interest began to flame between Harvey Cushing at Johns Hopkins, an increasingly visible figure, and those at the Harvard Medical School who supported his nomination as Surgeon-in-Chief. Prominent individuals provided him with consistent encouragement. As early as 1907, Dr. William Councilman, the Hopkins-trained Shattuck Professor of Pathological Anatomy at Harvard and one of Cushing's teachers wrote: "My dear Cushing: The Brigham Trustees have bought the land they need. Their general plans for the hospital have been agreed upon. So far as I know, you are the only man who would be considered for the place now."[13] Sir William Osler, a highly regarded teacher of several of the newly recruited faculty during their training at Johns Hopkins and one of Cushing's mentors, enthusiastically cabled from his lofty position as Regius Professor of Medicine at Oxford University, "Do Accept Harvard."[14] By 1911, despite other offers of surgical chairmanships around the country, the proposal had solidified to such an extent that J. Collins Warren, grandson of John Collins Warren of anesthesia fame, senior surgeon at the MGH, and the first Moseley Professor of Surgery at Harvard, was moved to exclaim: "I hear encouraging news about the Brigham Hospital and I am hoping some day when I go out to the medical school to rub my eyes and see a man with a spade in his hand."[15]

Despite such optimism, however, the languishing project evoked continuing frustration. The administration procrastinated regarding Cushing's appointment. "The [Harvard] corporation cannot be hurried. [President] Eliot is on the seas. The hospital trustees are slow and difficult. All of these folks are thinking but nothing is doing. Dr. Warren has resigned. No man can say what will be the outcome of it all."[16] Even when the young surgeon had moved to Boston a year later and had organized work in his new Surgical Research Laboratory in the medical school quadrangle, the clinical facilities remained incomplete.

Commensurate with the creation of any new institution, those in authority had to make a variety of decisions both important and trivial, as noted in the relevant correspondence of Francis B. Harrington and other decision makers. Perhaps as a retrospective illustration of enduring Boston medical nepotism, Harrington was the maternal grandfather of John Brooks, later to become an important member of the surgical faculty under Francis Moore and John Mannick, and the great-grandfather of David Brooks on the current surgical staff. A senior surgeon at the MGH, Harrington accepted the important position of external reviewer for many aspects of the planned hospital, including faculty and residency appointments, the workings of future departments, and an array of financial questions. For instance, he and H. M. Hurd, who had transferred from Hopkins to become the new Brigham superintendent, set the budget for the salaries of the entire hospital staff at $23,580. Department chairmen were to be offered $2,000–$5,000/year. "The professor of surgery, who has more opportunities for private work, [will] receive $3,000, two-thirds of which is paid by the hospital and one-third by the university."[17] The [chief] resident surgeon would receive $1,000 for the year; no other trainees were paid. And eventually they set the daily room rate for the patients at $15–$18, comparable to the 1910 charge of $17.50 per day that the MGH had raised from $16.52 in 1909.[18]

Involved directly in Cushing's appointment, Harrington describing the proposed terms in a letter to him in February 1910. "I have just had a talk with President Lowell [of Harvard]. From the conversation I feel safe in stating the following. If you accept the position of Surgeon-in-Chief of the Peter Bent Brigham Hospital you will at once be appointed Professor of Surgery and will be so designated in the publications of the University. Your active duties and your salary as Professor will begin as soon as you are ready to assume the work of teaching, whether at once or two years from now. Your functions in the School would not be subordinate to any other member of the Surgical Department and you would be expected to take the leading part in the future organization and development of the Surgical Instruction. In other words you would assume a position similar to the one now held by Dr. Maurice Richardson. Lowell's last remark to me was that he hoped to find in you a man who would do in your department here, what the leaders have done at Johns Hopkins in their departments."[19] There was no discussion about the Moseley Chair which Richardson, the senior surgeon at the MGH and its second incumbent, held. In fact, despite the initial concerns, Cushing assumed this position without difficulty as Richardson suddenly died before his arrival.

The Moseley Professorship of Surgery was initiated in 1898 and the Hersey Professorship in the Theory and Practice of Physic was endowed in 1792. Among the oldest and most prestigious academic chairs in the medical school, they were traditionally awarded to those at the MGH "because of its antiquity, its large clinics, and because of its high reputation."[20] Shortly after his appointment was confirmed, Cushing insisted that these titles be placed permanently at the Brigham as *the* university hospital. Despite President Lowell's objections to this change, the new professor won the rather protracted argument. As a result, he held one and Henry Christian, his counterpart in medicine and also Hopkins trained, the other. The chairs have resided at the Brigham since.

While the designated surgical chief was specific about demanding quality and training of nurses for their work in surgery and in the operating room, the subject of the formation of a Brigham nursing school provoked much administrative angst. In a letter to Harrington, the next superintendent, H. B. Howard, continued an apparently ongoing debate as to whether it should stand as a separate entity under its own head or be a part of the hospital hierarchy itself. His comments illustrate a well-established gender bias toward the latter arrangement.

"Last night you were speaking about the relative merits of an independent training school, and one that was really subordinate to the superintendent of the hospital, or better subordinate to the patients or the needs of the patients, who are in reality the hospital. I think that where the school is independent of the hospital and the training is merely sought as an end in itself, the patient's interests are sometimes lost sight of. The patient's welfare may receive due consideration but his comfort and happiness are a secondary consideration. If the ladies succeeded making that school independent it would rather belittle the [superintendent's] position. A strong independent man cannot be expected to still keep a position if you belittle his position. You have to get men to fill it who are little men and who can be pushed about, who will take one position one week and another the next. Mark my words, if the women of the training school get a man there to stand for having a superintendent of nurses independent of him, they will have a man that they themselves will not tolerate."[21]

The designated director of the nursing school and head nurse of the hospital, Carrie M. Hall, was an independent figure to reckon with. Her standards were high, her leadership firm but fair. In addition to her hospital and educational responsibilities, she organized nurses throughout Massachusetts into a Civil Defense Unit in the period leading up to World War I. For two years during the conflict itself, she headed the nursing unit of Harvard Base Hospital Number 5 in France. Decorated by several governments for her efforts, she was a match for many of the physicians around her and especially for Cushing. There was an ongoing "feud between her and Harvey Cushing: a feud albeit marked by mutual respect. During the ocean crossing writes Miss Hall, 'Dr. Cushing never spoke to me directly. If he wanted something, he would send [his assistant] Elliott Cutler to me. *I got along all right with him.*' "[22] An altercation that occurred in France in 1917 provoked a crisis that drove her to the written word. "My Dear Dr. Cushing: It is useless to try to evade the feeling of unpleasantness that exists between you and me. I cannot see my way clear to resigning [as Chief Nurse] except at your written request or at the request of the Red Cross." Needless to say, Miss Hall did not resign. After the war the "mutual respect" underlying their relationship lasted throughout their respective tenures.

With the opening of the hospital in 1913, personnel and patients slowly settled into place and Cushing began work. He and the individuals he gathered around him to staff the clinics and laboratories set a tone, tradition, esprit, and atmosphere of quality and inquiry that rarely faltered. From the beginning, the philosophy at "The Brigham" with its few faculty and modest bed capacity was different from the MGH, an older, larger, and grander sister institution across the city that had provided sympathetic and competent care for those seeking help for more than a century. Perhaps as a result it became heavily endowed through gifts from grateful patients and the sustained efforts of generations of trustees and supportive citizens. In contrast, the new enterprise with its modest size and limited bed capacity remained financially fragile, with talk of closure arising intermittently throughout much of its history. The numbers of the surgical and medical staff were limited. Relatively few residents were accepted into the highly competitive training programs. Gleaning as much physiological and pathological data as possible from each patient, the faculty and house staff all knew each other well, communicated easily and openly between their disciplines, and contributed jointly to ongoing innovations in the treatment of the ill.

11

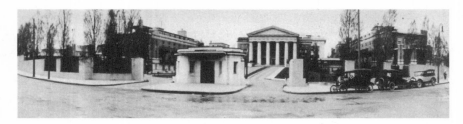

Figure 1.2   The entrance of the Peter Bent Brigham Hospital in 1920.

At cursory glance the new structure seemed a rather unlikely presence for what was to come. Adhering to traditional hospital design but generally contrasting with the more usual monolithic and multistory medical institutions arising in the United States, a series of "pavilions" were built based on the sanatorium concept of isolating infections and pestilence. The two-story brick and wooden buildings spread laterally. The "Pike," a 250-yard walkway with its south side draped with wisteria vines and open to the elements, was the backbone connecting the various wards and laboratories. Interestingly, John Shaw Billings,

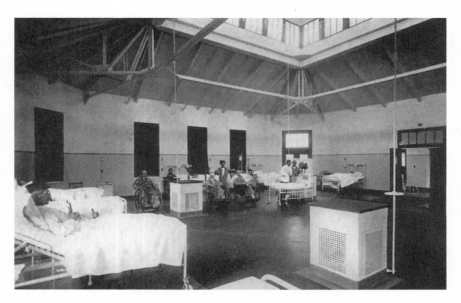

Figure 1.3   An open ward.

12

Surgeon-General of the Army, organizer of the *Index Medicus*, and driving force behind the creation of the Johns Hopkins Hospital, was also instrumental in the design of the Brigham.

But while the sprawling buildings lacked efficiency and cohesiveness, much about the arrangement was pleasant. Lawns, fruit trees, and a tennis court separated the circular, high ceilinged, 30-bed Nightingale wards that housed Mrs. Turner and the other "sick persons in indigent circumstances." Concrete floors beneath the beds "were heated to provide radiant energy and warmth. Each ward had several wide doorways through which beds could be pushed [outside]. Some patients were so enchanted with the open air, they came indoors only for nursing care or during severe weather."[23] Private patients on the second floor occupied individual cubicles divided by wooden partitions and with a curtain in front for privacy. When the weather was good they sunned themselves on the adjacent porches. It was different, however, during the colder months when the snow occasionally piled up along the Pike. Indeed, "the Brigham architect [who won a prize for his design of the building] has often been referred to as a man who never spent a winter in New England."[24] Some considered the new structure outdated and obsolete shortly after it was built.

One potential failing was lack of storage space. Billings had previously described a curious provision in the plans of the Hopkins Hospital that apparently was continued at the Brigham. "If a female nurse is a properly organized and healthy woman, she will certainly at times be subject to strong temptation, and this occurs in all hospitals where women are employed, without any exception whatever. Something may be done, however, to eliminate opportunities—and I believe, the [the lack of large closets] effects this as far as it is worth while to attempt it."[25] The source of "strong temptation," presumably the residents, was not mentioned.

Surrounded by classical columns, the front entrance led into a central rotunda. Doctor's offices opened off surrounding balconies. This large space was the social crossroads of the institution, housing the telephone switchboard, the reception desk, and the admitting and cashier's offices. A tall and stately matron, "Missus Carr, with a regal hairdo, a commanding voice, and an impressive bosom" managed the large semi-circular mahogany desk in the middle of the hall. "At 1 PM, she commandeered the four senior house officers to be available in the rotunda's lounge area for interviews with patients' visitors. It was a

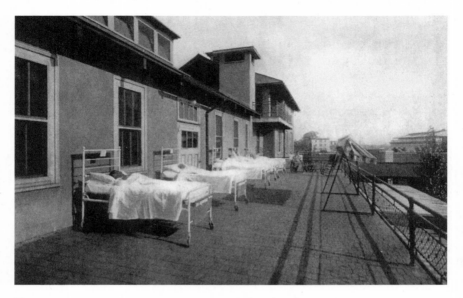

Figure 1.4   Patients sunning outside one of the private wards.

frenetic scene: visitors milled around each physician as the matron, dominating the melee, maintained order and made certain that each person had a chance to speak with the appropriate physician. Promptly at 2 PM she ordered the doors of the Pike opened, releasing a hundred or more visitors to make the noisy sprint to various bedsides. The rush was spectacular, particularly when the Pike was obscured by driving rain or buried in snow."[26]

During the day, an admitting nurse guided the patients to the appropriate doctor. At night, the telephone operator, Joe Connolly, operated the hospital switchboard from the desk behind which he sat in a reclining chair. A 10-foot cord plugged into the twin switchboards allowed him some latitude to wander. When the emergency doorbell sounded, he disconnected the cord and walked to a balcony overlooking the emergency entrance. Leaning over the wall, he shouted down to the person below. "'Be ye medical or be ye surgical? Have ye pain in the belly or ache in the heart? Are ye bloody?' With a perfunctory diagnosis, he trudged back to the switchboard, released the lock on the emergency room door, and once plugged back into the switchboard,

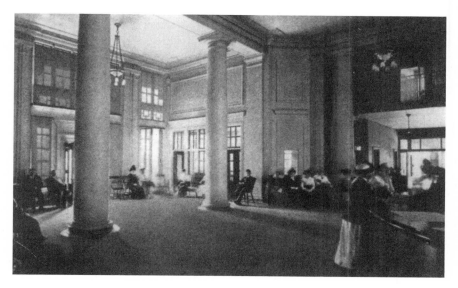

Figure 1.5   Inside the doors. The Rotunda.

summoned the appropriate house officer. If there was no response to the telephone, he resorted to the 'page', a hospital-wide system of resonant clappers." A Scottish Canadian, Joseph McQueen, superceded "Joe Front" in 1933. "Mac" not only kept the switchboard but checked assiduously that the students from the school of nursing made it back by curfew. He retired after nearly four decades.

The ambulance was another curious feature of the new hospital. "This was a large, black, cubic box fitted with wagon-like wheels with wooden spokes and hard rubber tires. A huge dish-shaped brass bell covered its left front door. A hand-operated brass hammer poised over its top edge always startled attention when needed. This 1913 electric vehicle was driven by either of two huge brothers who could barely crowd into the front seat. They took turns augmenting the electric power when a hill challenged the capacity of the antique batteries.

"Getting downhill posed a different problem. Speed had to be checked by dragging a piece of timber chained to the mid-frame of the ambulance as a chock for a rear wheel. A huge improvised brake lever controlled the length of chain. This extraordinary braking device persisted until 1939 when the ambulance was retired after a 'detailed

15

survey' showed it had made but 104 runs that year. Actually, conversion of the electric power supply of the hospital from DC to AC had robbed the ambulance of its battery charger."

By 1919, World War I was over. Lt. Colonel Cushing had returned from his duties in France. In his 6th *Annual Report of the Peter Bent Brigham Hospital,* he summarized the present status of his Department, discussing the familiar issues of providing excellent patient care, increasing the number of surgical operations, and the necessity for continued funding for the laboratory and the investigators within it. Of equal importance was his account of the visit of Sir William Osler to the new hospital on April 30, 1913 during his last lecture tour in North America.

"There hangs in the House Officers' dining room the first group picture taken in 1913, of the original band who came together to

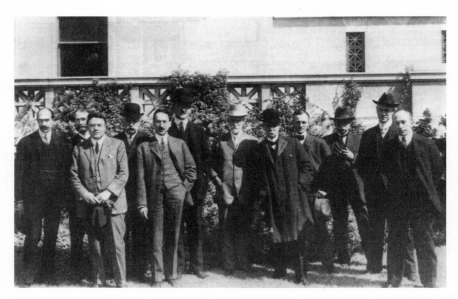

Figure 1.6   The opening of the new hospital, 1913. Left to right: John L. Bremer, Theobold Smith, Walter B. Cannon, Harold C. Ernst, Milton J. Rosenau, David L. Edsall, Charles S. Minot, Sir William Osler, Harvey Cushing, W.T. Councilman, Henry A. Christian, S. Burt Wolbach. From Aub JC, Hapgod RK, *Pioneer in Modern Medicine: David Linn Edsall* (Boston: Harvard Medical Alumni Assoc., 1970), 194.

constitute the professional, nursing, and administrative staff of the hospital. In the group were a few guests and the two central figures are John Collins Warren and William Osler, whose recent death has been felt so acutely by the entire medical profession. I have always thought of these two men as our guardian spirits of medicine and surgery.

"It happened that Sir William Osler was in the country on a visit and though we were in no condition to have a formal opening, his presence forced the occasion, for we wished his baptism even though the hospital was still in the stage of scaffolding and plaster. His influence, indeed, even without this early blessing of our venture was strong among us. His address to us which was taken down at the time was informal and not given with any expectation of publication, though it deserves reprinting in full. It is perhaps fitting at this time to recall some of his words."[27]

Osler's opening and closing statements were, Cushing recounted, as follows: "I have seen today what I have always wished would come here in Boston, what I have always thought would come; I have seen a new and perfectly striking departure in hospital growth. You are part of a great organization, you are taking a very important step in medical education, and this is a great thing for the city and for the country in the future development of medicine." With Osler's blessing, the new enterprise was launched.

CHAPTER 2

HARVEY CUSHING
AND THE MAKING OF
AN ACADEMIC SURGEON

F EW SURGEONS IN modern history have left behind such a trail of relevant information as Harvey Cushing. Indeed, his accomplishments were so broad and interests so diverse that biographers for years have recorded his activities and kept alive his memory. The quantity and quality of his writings has made their task easier. A prolific correspondent, keeper of diaries, and collector of family papers even at a young age, he expanded these talents during his life through his copious professional and literary contributions. His primary biographer, John Fulton, believed that Cushing wrote 10,000 words each day during his 20-year tenure as Surgeon-in-Chief at the Brigham. One of his successors, Francis Moore, calculated that his daily output was 40 typewritten pages, excluding drafts, adding wryly that to produce his biography all Fulton had to do was "simply put all this together end-to-end."[1] Never one to underestimate his own abilities, fame, and legacy, Cushing may have produced these effusions with an eye toward his later immortality.

HE WAS BORN INTO a distinguished and somewhat ascetic medical family. His father was a successful physician in Cleveland; his grandfather and great-grandfather had been doctors in Massachusetts. His older brother, Ned, an ebullient and cheerful individual rather different from the other more austere male family members, may have attracted his sibling toward those of similar temperament and stimulated him toward a more conscious use of his often hidden but not inconsiderable charm. Migrating eastward to Yale University, Cushing immediately became caught up in college life probably to the detriment of his academic record. Indeed, his biographers have all remarked upon his reputedly slow intellectual development. But the strong attachment he formed with his college, based primarily on extra-curricular pleasures, lasted all his life. He reminisced on this subject years later. "The library on the western boundary of the old campus was to us merely a building and not a collection of animate books, the necessary tools of education. I remember once and only once—taking a look within its gloomy portal and wondering how anyone could choose to waste the all too fleeting days of youth in that gloomy place, where Lux was dim and Veritas had the musty smell of moldering calf. We passed much of the next four years sweating in the old Gym to qualify for our chosen forms of sport."[2]

His enthusiasm toward his chosen forms of sport, particularly varsity baseball, burgeoned despite warnings from his rather puritanical father. "The convictions I hold concerning college games and contests are no less strong than when you left home. Indeed, the more I hear of them, the more settled do I become in my belief that they are an evil of the first magnitude."[3] Dr. Cushing continued in this tone in a follow-up letter after discovering that his son actually intended to play against Harvard: "I will try to reply to your letter calmly, though I do feel sore and disturbed over the unhappy position you have brought us into. I carefully explained before you went to New Haven that we were going into a partnership with mutual responsibilities and duties. I was to supply the means, and you to conduct yourself to my approval while the partnership survived. Among the conditions I insisted on and which I understood you to assent to, were that you would not smoke, drink or be guilty of any immoral conduct or joining a College ball club or boat crew."[4] Suffice it to say, not only did Cushing begin to smoke but played baseball creditably throughout his undergraduate years.

His fondness for Yale lasted all his life and fostered his return to New Haven during his retirement. "He found Yale a congenial and pleasant place for the expression of [his] three remarkable traits of inner drive, influence by elders, and peer group friendships, all three of them, evident [throughout] his career."[5]

Despite the blandishments of the athletic and social life, his interest in science and ultimately in medicine became focused enough that he followed his brother Ned to Harvard Medical School in 1891, entering the final three-year class. Although the faculty had improved substantially since President Eliot had reorganized the school and revamped its hitherto languishing curriculum, there is little to suggest that Cushing enjoyed the experience. However, his leadership traits and technical abilities, manifested particularly in the dissection of cadavers, were becoming recognized. His first 'part' was a right arm. Before long the instructors and his fellow students were watching the dissection. Set apart from his peers by this display and realizing the significance of his talents, he began to devote himself resolutely to his future surgical career.

His early clinical experience at the MGH as a medical student ranged between the amusing and the depressing, as well as influencing some of his later interests. In a letter to his father, for instance, he wrote: "yesterday, my out-patient engagement wound up. I don't know how much I have learned there except to ask people with more or less grace—'how are your bowels?' One good old creature told me his were in Ireland. I presume he didn't quite catch the drift of my question."[6]

A devastating experience occurred with the administration of anesthesia when Cushing was a third-year student. "My first giving of an anesthetic was when I was called down from the seats and sent into a little side room with the patient and an orderly and told to put the patient to sleep. I knew nothing about the patient whatsoever, merely the nurse came in and gave him a hypodermic injection. I proceeded as best I could under the orderly's directions and in view of the repeated calls from the amphitheater it seemed to me an interminable time for the old man, who kept gagging, to go to sleep. We finally wheeled him in. I can vividly recall, even now, just how he looked and the feel of his bedraggled whiskers. The operation was started and at this juncture there was a sudden great gush of fluid from the patient's mouth, most of that was inhaled, and he died. I stood aside, burning with chagrin and remorse. No one paid the slightest attention to me, although I supposed that I had killed the patient. I slunk out of the Hospital, walked the streets of North Boston the rest of the afternoon, and in the evening went to the surgeon's house to ask if there was any possible way I could atone for the calamity of the man's family before I left the medical school and went into some other business. To my perfect amazement I was told it was nothing at all, that I had nothing to do with the man's death, that he had a strangulated hernia and had been vomiting all night anyway, and that sort of thing happened frequently and I had better forget about it and go on with medical school. I went on with the medical school but I have never forgotten about it."[7]

While death under anesthesia at that time was "nothing at all," Cushing felt that this was a situation he could improve. Within two years he and a classmate, Ernest Amory Codman, devised an ether chart as a precise record of the patient's respirations and pulse rate. Codman went on to emphasize that hospital organization of the time was inferior, creating standards which led to the modern morbidity and mortality conference, the classification of complications or deaths in regard to whether they were on the basis of physician error or from the processes of disease, and a general increase in the quality of patient care. As an unwelcome prophet in his own time, he generated much antipathy among his peers.

Cushing later rekindled these early interests in patient monitoring by bringing back a Riva-Rocci blood pressure apparatus from Italy in 1901 and requiring its use during all his subsequent surgical procedures. As this new concept provoked attention in at least one distant city, professors at Harvard formed a committee to study it. After lengthy deliberation, the *Harvard Blood Pressure Circular* appeared which asserted dogmatically that "the skilled finger was of much greater value clinically for determination of the state of the circulation than any pneumatic instrument."[8] Within a few years, needless to say, the "pneumatic instrument" was in general use, consistently outperforming "the skilled finger."

A rotation in the psychiatric division of a nursing home outside Boston during his final year of medical school may have directed his attention toward the workings of the central nervous system, providing him contact with neurologic and psychiatric patients as well as exposure to occasional operations on the brain. His internship at the MGH in 1895 and his initial experience at Johns Hopkins a year later brought him into contact with similar patients. One who particularly impressed the young trainee presented shortly after he started his surgical residency at Hopkins. Lizzie W. had been shot in the neck by her husband, a bartender. The development of a classic Brown-Sequard Syndrome, with lack of sensation on one side of her body below the injury, allowed Cushing to deduce the location of the bullet which had lodged in her spine. As he and Codman had investigated the potential clinical usefulness of the new technique of roentgenography the year before in

Boston, and as he had continued studies with a fluoroscope that he had brought with him to Baltimore, he demonstrated accurately the location of the bullet in the sixth cervical vertebra. His careful and accurate mapping of the full extent of her neurological defects during her six-month stay became the subject of his first publication.[9]

Important advances were revolutionizing surgery and surgical care by the middle of the nineteenth century. The first was the control of sepsis after childbirth by understanding that a physician or nurse could spread contamination to healthy patients and that simple hygiene could prevent it. In 1865, a surgeon in Glasgow, Joseph Lister, produced another critical improvement. Up to that time, few patients survived an operation unscathed. Instruments were rarely cleaned between cases. Surgeons operated in pus- and blood-encrusted frock coats, with ligatures hanging from a buttonhole for use during the procedure. Under such conditions, operative sites often became septic. Sepsis often led to death. Based on the observation that phenol killed contaminating bacteria and from the corroborating evidence from gypsies who had used the material to cleanse wounds for generations, Lister began to operate in a continuous spray of phenol-containing "carbolic acid," an antiseptic solution that enveloped surgeon, patient, and the surgical field alike. Despite antipathy to the concept in the United States, it gradually gained acceptance and was improved further by the principle of asepsis, the sterilization of instruments, surgical gowns, and other accoutrements, as well as total cleanliness of the operating room.

Regardless of such progress, one should remember that even during Cushing's training 20 years later, no masks were worn, rubber gloves had just been introduced but not accepted by all, spectators wearing street clothes often crowded the operating rooms, and many aspects of surgical techniques now taken for granted were not yet in place. Operations to drain appendiceal abscesses or opening the gall bladder to remove stones were just becoming routine. A description of the surgical methods at the MGH in 1889, only a few years before his internship, is instructive. "The peritoneal cavity was opened only for emergencies, such as bleeding gastric ulcer or intestinal obstruction. Operations on the gall bladder, spleen, or kidney were very infrequent. Much of the surgery was done in a dense fog of carbolic spray. Solutions of carbolic acid or bichloride of mercury were used freely to irri-

gate wounds. Drainage tubes were inserted after almost every operation. A wound that healed without pus formation was a matter of comment. The surgeon and his assistants washed their hands with soap and
water and rinsed them in bichloride or carbolic acid solution. The surgeons did not wear clean white suits. Operating coats were covered
with spots of blood and pus, and were rarely cleaned. No wonder sup-
purating wounds and drainage tubes were the order of the day."[10]
Indeed, sterilization of instruments with dry heat was considered a
novelty.

Anesthesia was an equally important development. Before it became
available, operations were a last and dreaded resort. The operating theater was a torture chamber where surgical procedures were carried out
on screaming and struggling patients. A gas, nitrous oxide, had been
known since the end of the eighteenth century to produce pleasurable
sensations, particularly laughter, among those who breathed it. Occasionally they became unconscious and appeared impervious to the
effects of injury. Only decades later did some in the medical profession,
particularly in the United States, consider seriously that the substance
might be used advantageously in surgery. A dentist from Hartford,
Horace Wells, first experienced its anesthetic effects in 1844, having
convinced a colleague to pull one of his molar teeth under its influence.
Unfortunately, his subsequent public demonstration was a failure.
About the same time, a rural Georgia practitioner, Crawford Long,
noted that another gas, ether, dulled the pain of injury. A young Boston
dentist, William Morton, upstaged Long in 1846 at the MGH by using
the agent so convincingly that the surgeon, John Collins Warren, ligated a large vascular anomaly in the neck of one Edward Abbott calmly
and without producing pain. The coincident successful experience in
Britain with chloroform in childbirth cemented this new concept into
general use. And Queen Victoria, who had received it during some of
her own deliveries, approved.

WITH SURGEONS INCREASINGLY ACCEPTING the critical innovations
of anesthesia, antisepsis, and asepsis by the opening of the twentieth
century, operative interventions broadened in scope and variety. Fundamental changes in the teaching of surgery and the surgical sciences
also gained momentum, stimulated in large part by the model pro-
ferred by the Johns Hopkins Medical School and its Hospital. Surgical
education became more relevant and practical as the instructors

migrated from amphitheater to bedside. Students spent more time on the wards caring for the patients. Increasingly, comprehensive medical school courses familiarized elective students with technical details of surgery and anatomy, surgical pathology and histology. Following demonstration of specific operative procedures, the students would repeat them on cadavers under the critical eye of their preceptors.

William Stewart Halsted, one of the foremost surgeons of the time and the newly-named chief of surgery at Hopkins was responsible for many of these improvements. A meticulous technician and surgical innovator who adhered strictly to anatomical and physiological principles, he surrounded himself with a succession of highly talented residents. After many years of formal training under his aegis, they spread his philosophy, standards, and methods throughout the country.

Cushing became a devoted disciple. Although he spent his internship year at the MGH, he had become so impressed with the surgical program at Hopkins during a visit with his brother Ned that he applied for a residency position. After an apparently prolonged dialogue, Halsted finally accepted him into his program. Indeed, there was debate as to whether he would be chosen at all. In a April 1896 letter replying to his request for a position, Halsted noted: "I am sorry to have to tell you that beginning with the next Spring it is to be our policy to fill all the places on the staff of the Johns Hopkins Hospital with graduates of the Johns Hopkins Medical School. If you care for a place on my staff before next fall, I can probably give it to you. This is as much as I can promise anyone who has not worked with me."[11]

While Cushing had enjoyed his time at the MGH and held several of the surgeons there in high esteem, he was less enthusiastic about some of the others: "Not operating much. Considerable sepsis in the house. No wonder, these men operate about the way a commercial traveler grabs breakfast at the lunch counter."[12] His opinions about the teaching were equally critical. "We operated too much by the clock: the wealth of material was utilized in no way except for added experiences: cases were insufficiently studied before operation. We disdained the students, forgetting how recently we had been one of them; there was rather too much display and operative rivalry at a Saturday morning public exhibition of skills; too much of the week's hard work was postponed for a prolonged Sunday morning visit which left us with no day of relaxation. There was no spur whatever to perfection; no encouragement to follow up the bad result."[13]

In contrast, Halsted's careful operative techniques impressed him greatly. Elliott Cutler, Cushing's successor at the Brigham, later exemplified the differences between the Baltimore and Boston surgical philosophies. "The shift from the Boston surgery of the day, where speed of operating was still considered advisable and even used as a gauge for ability, to the painstaking, slow and gentle methods of Halsted was an everlasting inspiration to the pupil Cushing. He often told the story himself that, coming from Boston where a complete breast procedure was accomplished in 28 minutes, he saw with misgiving a four and one half-hour operation for the same undertaking. How amazed he was that stimulants were unnecessary and how horrified he was when told not to dress the wound for ten days! Recalling the wounds he had previously studied, he remarked to himself: 'I may not see the wound, but I will smell it!' When in ten days the wound was dressed and found perfectly healed, his skepticism disappeared. Moreover, here he was first introduced to the experimental method and was taught the value of careful and detailed records whether in the laboratory or on the ward. From Halsted, he learned that precise and thorough concentration on a small problem might yield more than great labors in routine work. Here, too, he learned the value of a meticulous and gentle technique that sought to spare each cell from being damaged, a technique which was to permit him later to operate on the central nervous system. It is doubtful if Halsted had any other trainees who learned so rapidly and thoroughly the art of surgical procedures as he, Halsted, conceived it."[14]

Cushing became Halsted's chief surgical resident, the fifth of seventeen who ultimately achieved that exalted rank. Carrying out many general surgical procedures, his widening clinical experience, striking technical abilities, and single-minded determination contributed to his increasing reputation. He became the first surgeon in the United States to perform splenectomy for Banti's syndrome, the twelfth case in the world. Characteristically, he followed this patient for 40 years, eventually writing him to congratulate him on his fourth marriage. Becoming interested in peripheral nerve anesthesia with cocaine, unaware of the significant and ongoing problems that Halsted had with the addictive substance, and perhaps still equivocal about the safety of general anesthesia, Cushing developed local techniques for hernia repair, amputations, and other operations.[15] He was also responsible for a large surgical clinic.

During this period and in the decade to come, he investigated a variety of subjects that involved the results of general surgical procedures and the importance of electrolytes in patient homeostasis. He became expert in surgical bacteriology, having accrued experience with closure of intestinal perforations secondary to typhoid fever during and after the Spanish-American War.[16] These studies brought him into contact with such bacteriological notables as Theobald Smith, Simon Flexner, and Walter Reed who were also studying the paratyphoid organism. His growing interests in neurosurgery also became evident despite little encouragement from those around him. An early neurosurgical paper appeared in print eight days after he had presented an innovative surgical approach at the College of Physicians of Philadelphia to treat trigeminal neuralgia by ablating the Gasserian ganglion, perhaps a record for rapid publication.[17] He was 31 years old when he finished his residency at Hopkins. With this background, his future was becoming focused.

In addition to his heavy clinical load, Cushing began to develop other passions. Encouraged by his evolving friendship with William Osler and influenced by Osler's enthusiastic bibliophilia, he became increasingly interested in rare medical books, bookplates, and forming the beginnings of a library. Other Hopkins mentors further kindled these enthusiasms. Halsted gave him 25 volumes of the transactions of the German Surgical Society, and William Kelly, the professor of obstetrics at Hopkins, even more generously presented him with a superb copy of a 1555 edition of Vesalius's *De Humani Corporis Fabrica*.

Within a few years his book collecting had taken on a deeper intellectual value for him than just adding another volume to his shelves.[18] He described the appetites of the book lover in 1903. "A friend has been staying with me whose metabolism and pulse rate in the presence of other people's books run high. So while you endeavor to concentrate upon your proper tasks he exclaims, 'Where did you get this Dolet imprint?' holding up a vaguely remembered calf of a book in his hand. 'Are you aware that Christie only knew of one other copy?' This is enough; you are lost. The attack of influenza is nothing to it, and days elapse before you are fit to resume your legitimate job. *Beware the book!*"[19]

He broadened his outlook further by meeting the eminent in his field and working with prominent scientists during a 14-month sojourn in Europe at the beginning of the new century. Never one to eschew personal contacts, he cultivated friendships and acquaintances during these wanderings and gained surgical and neurosurgical role models. These included Theodor Kocher in Berne, one of the few surgeons to win the Nobel Prize for his work on the physiology, pathology, and surgery of the thyroid gland, and Sir Victor Horsley, a neurosurgical pioneer in London. Although this latter friendship gave him great pleasure, he was less impressed by Horsley's operative techniques.

"He found [him] sitting in seemingly great confusion; dictating letters during breakfast to male secretaries; patting dogs between letters; and operating like a wild man. HC gave him a reprint of his paper on the Gasserian ganglion, whereupon Horsley said he would show him how to do a case. They drove off the next morning in Horsley's cab, after sterilizing the instruments in Horsley's house and packing them in a towel, to a well-appointed West End mansion. Horsley dashed upstairs, had his patient under ether in five minutes and was operating 15 minutes after he entered the house; he made great holes in the woman's skull, pushing up the temporal lobe—blood everywhere, gauze packed into the middle fossa, the ganglion cut, the wound closed, and he was out of the house in less than an hour after he entered it. This experience settled Cushing's decision to leave London; for he felt that the refinements of neurological surgery could not be learned from Horsley."[20]

The productivity and spirit of the continental laboratories of physiology that he visited and the encouragement of his preceptors had been so stimulating to the young investigator that he found himself increasingly devoted to the study of neurological disease, its manifestations and its surgical correction. But as his interest in the subject burgeoned, his colleagues felt that he was grasping at shadows, particularly as the occasional operations for cerebral tumors and other central conditions were almost invariably unsuccessful. Indeed, the few attempts had been disastrous. Surgeons rarely dared to expose the brain by dividing its covering membranes until well after the routine acceptance of asepsis. Infection seemed inevitable. Although they occasionally elevated depressed fractures of the skull, removed adjacent blood clots, repaired lacerations of the scalp, and drained superficial abscesses, they considered relatively little else. Most importantly, means to localize abnormalities within the skull were rudimentary. While physical examination was of some help, diagnostic tools were limited to crude and inadequate cranial x-rays. Autopsy confirmed their inadequacies. Horseley's neurological colleagues in London, aghast at the mortality rate, sent him cases as a last resort. Kocher, a master surgeon, had undertaken only one operation on the brain. He had to retreat promptly because of massive and uncontrollable bleeding.

Joining the Johns Hopkins surgical staff upon his return from the continent, Cushing requested the opportunity to work in the then virtually unrecognized field of neurosurgery. The prospects were worse than he realized. Indeed, during the decade of existence of the hospital, the diagnosis of brain tumor had been made only 32 times among the 36,000 patients admitted. Thirteen individuals with that diagnosis had been transferred to surgery; two had been operated upon disastrously. Most of the remainder had their diagnosis confirmed after death.[21] And Halsted skeptically noted that only two cases of brain tumor were referred for operation in the last year. But after further pressing and despite encouragement to enter orthopedics, Cushing endured and the field was his.

Busy, active, and enormously productive as a young member of Halsted's department, his character could be difficult and often arrogant. A perfectionist from an early age, his compulsive and meticulous nature was evident in all facets of his life, from changing surgical dressings to his literary output. Thin, intense, and hard driving, he enjoyed scheduling complex operations or dressing changes on holidays or weekends to keep the house staff alert. Years later one of his fellow trainees at the MGH described these youthful personality traits. "He was recognized as perhaps the ablest man in his class at the Medical School and was an extremely hard worker. As House Officer, I was his junior and suffered extremely in that position for a year. He was an extremely hard man to work with, whether one was over him or under him, as his tremendous ambition for success made it impossible for him to allow anyone else to get any credit for work done. When he wanted to be he was one of the most charming people in the world, but working with him I found that he couldn't tolerate anyone else in the limelight."[22]

His prodigious energies and compulsive manner did not make life easy either for his residents or for some of his faculty colleagues. Perhaps influenced by his own research experience with the authoritarian figure of Kocher who had virtually ignored his young visitor until he believed him to be a serious student, Cushing considered that those on the house staff who could not withstand his treatment were unsuitable for the rigors of later surgical practice. Most stayed. Occasionally during his early tenure at Hopkins, however, even Osler had to pull on the reins regarding his interactions with others. "The statement is correct that you do not get on well with your surgical subordinates and colleagues. Keep your mouth (as the Psalmist says) as it were with a bridle."[23]

While the early results of surgery on the nervous system were discouraging and the mortality rate high, Cushing's careful operative dissections, compulsive patient follow-up, and precise evaluation of postmortem findings gradually improved his successes. Ideas sprouted from clinical conundrums. From the bedside and from the laboratory came a ferment of activity examining and defining both normal and abnormal physiology of the central nervous system and its interactions with the endocrine glands.

Realizing well his technical abilities, Cushing summarized his thoughts about behavior in the operating room in a 1913 address. "The accurate and detailed methods, in the use of which Kocher and Halsted were for so long the notable examples, have spread into all clinics—at least into those clinics where you or I would wish to entrust ourselves for operation. Observers no longer expect to be thrilled in an operating room; the spectacular public performances of the past, no longer condoned, are replaced by the quiet, rather tedious procedures which few beyond the operator, his assistants, and the immediate bystander can profitably see. The patient on the table, like the passenger in a car, runs greater risks if he has a loquacious driver, or one who takes close corners, exceeds the speed limit, or rides to admiration."[24]

Although research was another of Cushing's lifelong commitments, its pursuit was not only unusual for young doctors of the time but rarely presented as part of their surgical education. But without this novel discipline it is doubtful that much progress in modern surgery would have occurred. Pragmatic surgeons designing experimental models in the laboratory to answer questions arising at the bedside have consistently produced new knowledge and continuing advances in patient care throughout much of the twentieth century.

Cushing's scientific experiences in Europe had stimulated his interest in applied investigations. Joining the laboratory of the experimental physiologist, Hugo Kronecker in Berne, he examined two questions, the systemic effects of raising intracranial pressure and the influence of electrolyte ions on muscle physiology. In dogs, he showed that increased intracranial tension caused systolic blood pressure to rise, a response later recognized clinically as "the Cushing effect."[25] In frogs, he demonstrated that sodium chloride inhibited muscular activity but that addition of small amounts of potassium could restore normal responsiveness.[26] Moving on to Liverpool, he worked with the physiologist Charles Scott Sherrington who was mapping the motor cortex of the three great anthropoid apes, chimpanzee, gorilla, and orangutan. Cushing's line drawings eventually appeared in one of Sherrington's publications.[27] A burgeoning friendship with the pioneer endocrinologist, Alfred Fröhlich, whetted his growing interest in the pituitary and neuroendocrine system. His overall experience with these well-known investigators influenced substantially his thinking about surgical education and the later organization of his own residency program. "I acquired more of real value for my surgical work [in these laboratories] than in my previous six years of service as hospital intern."[28]

The subject of experimental biology carried out in living animals had arisen early in the nineteenth century in France and Germany as a means to understand normal bodily functions and dysfunctions based on pathological conditions, and to define and answer questions regarding actual mechanisms of disease.[29] In Britain, the subject remained of relatively minor concern, as much of the medical establishment was loath to accept the importance of laboratory research over the traditionally strong clinical subjects of physical diagnosis and human anatomy. In the 1870s, however, the field transformed into an increasingly powerful force when eminent investigators opened research institutes. About the same time, the Royal College of Surgeons began to demand more specialized knowledge about the normal behavior and function of the body by those taking their qualifying examinations. Medical schools started their own laboratories and recruited physiologists to direct them.

In the United States, the concept of a surgical laboratory that involved the teaching of operative techniques to students and the solving of clinical problems in animals began as a new departure from established traditions. Only two were started. Halsted had introduced the first and only course in experimental surgery in 1895 to teach and explore operative techniques. He elaborated on this theme in a published description of his method of joining the ends of the intestine after a portion had been removed, one of his lasting contributions to surgery. "I should be sorry to have it forgotten that I initiated the operative course on animals. Courses in experimental surgery were given to the first class in their third year."[30] He credited his younger colleagues with the success of the venture, particularly Cushing. "In our laboratory operative courses for students, the leading topic from the time of the introduction of these exercises, has been intestinal suture. I embrace this opportunity to express my indebtedness to Harvey Cushing, for thirteen years my brilliant assistant, for his zeal in elaborating these courses and placing them on such a substantial basis that they are now regarded as one of the dominant features of the surgical curriculum and are being adopted by other medical schools of this country."

In 1901, J. Collins Warren opened a surgical laboratory at Harvard, the second in the country. At that time, no single director or consultant was available to advise laboratory workers or to supervise individual research projects, as medical school traditions encouraged young surgeons to involve themselves with morphology and dissection rather than physiology and the experimental method. Warren instituted a journal in 1903, *The HMS Department of Surgery Bulletin*, for young investigators to report their research results, hoping that it would stimulate interest in scientific investigations and enhance a proper laboratory of experimental surgery. He stated his aims in his first report. "The following papers are presented by the Surgical Department of the HMS as evidence of its ambition to encourage original work and to train men for research in the many branches of surgery and surgical pathology. We have been able to make a marvelous beginning with funds at present in possession, derived partly from small endowments and partly from annual gifts. The enthusiasm and capacity exhibited by the young men of this Department for investigations of this character, is most encouraging and it is confidently expected that with the almost ideal facilities which are to be given in the new building for the medical school, they will not be wanting, and be worthy of the occasion. The new quarters for surgical research have been planned with the greatest care and are on a scale that leaves nothing to be desired—except a suitable endowment. We cannot refrain from expressing great confidence in the belief that when the importance of the work in which we are engaged has been made clear to the public, generous patrons will be found willing to place this part of our labors upon an enduring basis."[31] Subjects under investigation included cesarean section, atrophy following joint fixation, surgery involving lung, arteries, spleen, and ureters, production and prevention of peritoneal adhesions, and intestinal lavage.

Responsibility for an elective surgical anatomy course was one of the inducements that Halsted offered his young protégé to return to the Hopkins staff. This included both a series of lectures to the third-year medical students and a practical session in operative technique using both cadavers and animals. Although Halsted's original course in experimental surgery had been set up as demonstrations to small groups of students, Cushing quickly expanded its breadth and improved its popularity and value to such an extent that it became dominant in the surgical curriculum. He expected the students to organize and pack supplies, select and sterilize instruments, and perform operations on dogs to simulate as closely as possible actual procedures carried out in patients. They administered anesthesia, wrote a history and peri-operative and postoperative notes, kept an ether chart during the surgery, made rounds thereafter, and performed a postmortem examination if the animal died.

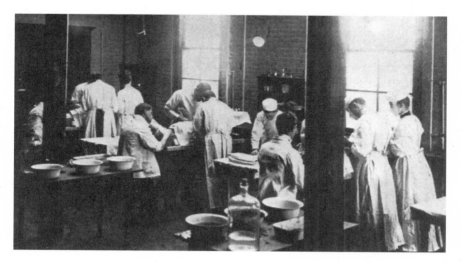

FIGURE 2.1   The Old Hunterian Laboratory at Johns Hopkins in 1910. From Crowe SJ, *Halsted of Johns Hopkins: the Man and His Men* (Springfield: Charles C. Thomas, 1957), 70.

Because of increasing enrollment in the dog course and lack of space for any coincident investigative work in the existing facilities at the Johns Hopkins Hospital, plans for a new laboratory were instituted. Cushing described the circumstances years later: "During the year, I believe 1904, W. G. MacCallum [Professor of Pathology] who had found that the facilities in the pathological building were inadequate for the type of experimental work he was interested in entered into a conspiracy with me and together we made another appeal, which this time was backed up by the students, for a simple building which we could utilize for experimental work—and which could serve as a center for all the animals utilized by the school. To our great gratification our plans were accepted and during the year 1905, the 'Old Hunterian' was erected, I believe at a cost of $15,000. We had a good deal of discussion as to what the laboratory ought to be called. I was in favor of naming it the Magendie laboratory [pioneer nineteenth century French experimental physiologist] although the anti-vivisection group in Baltimore was very active at the time and François Magendie's name was anathema to them. So, with the suggestion of Dr. Welch, we thought we would use John Hunter's [the great eighteenth century experimental surgeon] name instead—hence the Hunterian Laboratory of Experimental Medicine.

"It was not a bad solution for it mystified a good many people who thought that the term had something to do with a pointer or a setter, and after all it did have something to do with them for we began to have a good deal of veterinary work."[32]

Cushing's course not only provided practical teaching of surgical techniques but stimulated contacts between students and their teachers that often led to the investigation of various topics. He targeted a few likely individuals at the end of each session to participate in research projects involving canine morbid physiology and comparative pathology. He then invited the best students to apply for a surgical residency. Because of his growing clinical responsibilities, he also appointed an assistant from among the residents to run the Hunterian Laboratory for a year, a pattern that presaged the organization of his laboratory at Harvard. The chosen individual had to possess good scholastic qualifications, enthusiasm for research, and the ability to work alone. During his time in charge, the incumbent was to devote himself primarily to laboratory studies generally oriented toward the neurological sciences. The following year would be spent on his clinical service. Any pub-

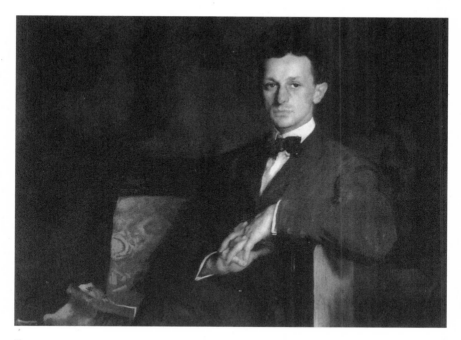

Figure 2.2   Harvey Cushing, portrait by Edmund C. Tarbell, 1908 (Dittrick Medical History Center, with permission).

lishable material was to be written in collaboration with Cushing. His efforts and those of his disciples, combined with more formal operative instruction and the availability of human cadavers to allow students to undertake specific procedures, produced fundamental changes in the teaching of surgery and surgical sciences that many medical schools would also soon initiate.

As may happen in any institution in which a superior staff stimulates its own and each other's productivity, the contributions of the surgeons at Johns Hopkins in the early twentieth century were legion. Halsted had originally performed experiments with intestinal suture and techniques of vascular anastomosis. His studies on the physiology of the thyroid and parathyroid glands complimented those of Hopkins pathologists who had noted the relationship between parathyroid function and calcium metabolism. Under Cushing, research fellows began to study the influence of the internal secretion of the pancreas on carbohydrate metabolism and noted, with a few other investigators of the time, that diabetes mellitus ensued following removal of the gland. They studied experimental hydrocephalus and devised the technique of ventriculography, an important contribution to neurosurgery. These and other advances produced by individuals working in the Old Hunterian acted as a bellwether not only for the surgical laboratory at Harvard, but in the laboratories formed subsequently in other medical schools in the United States.

CHAPTER 3

THE PROFESSOR AND HIS BRIGHAM CAREER

TRANSCENDING the bleak beginnings of the new field, Cushing became recognized as the pioneer neurosurgeon of the country within a few years of his new appointment. But he had expended much effort during his time in Baltimore to achieve this prominence. As noted, he published a landmark article on removing the Gasserian ganglion while still a resident in 1900, having first practiced his technique assiduously on cadavers in the anatomy laboratory.[1] Five years later he presented a second report of 20 such cases, describing each patient in detail, defining the surgical indications for the procedure, characterizing the sub-temporal approach, and analyzing the results.[2] He carried out these and other operations on the central nervous system, it must be recalled, during a time of rudimentary radiology, infrequent blood transfusions, or even the general availability of white blood cell counts. His 1908 chapter on cranial surgery in William Williams Keen's eight-volume *Surgery, Its Principles and Practice* added substantially to his reputation and acted as a catalyst for the future growth of the subject in the United States. Indeed, after many negotiations with the publisher he reduced his huge treatise from 800 pages to a monograph of 276 pages with 154 illustrations. The chapter was reprinted by the Surgeon General as a handbook on traumatic injury of the head for use by the Army during World War I.

With broadening experience, an increasing caseload, and an improving success rate, he became increasingly interested in the pituitary gland and its functions. In 1901, a 16-year-old girl presented to Dr. Osler with headaches, failing vision, stunted growth, and underdeveloped secondary sexual characteristics. Although suspecting that a pituitary tumor had caused these changes, Cushing was unable to locate it during three separate surgical explorations. At autopsy, the tumor lay in the anterior lobe of the gland. About the same time and to his chagrin, he received a letter from Fröhlich describing a similar patient who had been operated on successfully in Europe. In 1908, Professor Edward Sharpey-Schafer, a well-known Scottish physiologist and colleague of Horsley, provoked his enthusiasm further by a series of lectures on the subject.

Desirous of understanding the gland more fully, the young neurosurgeon directed John Homans and other research fellows working in the Old Hunterian Laboratory to examine the effects of its removal in dogs. One of the investigators described the experiments: "This work was done under the supervision of Doctor Cushing, who always came to the laboratory every afternoon after he had finished his day's work in the hospital. It was on one of these visits that we told him about a female fox terrier that we had operated on 92 days previously. At this operation the pituitary stalk was divided, and in addition a portion of the anterior lobe removed. On that day of the operation (December 18, 1908) the animal weighed 14 pounds. Following the operation there was a rapid gain in weight from 14 to 24 pounds, and six months later there had been no sign that the dog had been in heat since the operation. Doctor Cushing looked over the notes we had made on this animal, and asked that she be brought up so that he could see her. After taking one look he became very much excited and said 'This is Frölich's asexual adiposity, experimentally produced.' This was about five o'clock. It was hours before we got home that night."[3]

Cushing discussed his thinking about the subject. "There had long been great confusion as to whether acromegaly, Frölich's syndrome and so on were expressions of over or underactivity of the gland. Frölich, as you will remember, reported his case as one of tumor of the pituitary body without acromegaly, the implications being that it was astonishing a tumor of the pituitary could occur without acromegaly. The first definite indication that the syndrome of Frölich and other allied syndromes were due to an hypophyseal insufficiency, was furnished by the experiments conducted with Homans."

He began increasingly to realize that the "master gland" controlled all endocrine activity and conceptualized that if Froelich's Syndrome occurred secondary to a lack of glandular secretions, growth abnormalities such as giantism must be due to oversecretion. Accruing understanding of the overall role of this critical organ allowed progressively accurate assessment of its various functions, fifty years before precise chemical methods for determining its hormones in the blood became available.

His interest in individuals afflicted with pituitary abnormalities also caused him to spend time at the circus, locating, meeting and examining giants, dwarfs, and those with sexual immaturity. "Cushing's work on the pituitary made him particularly aware and sympathetic with the abnormal conditions which so often found their way to the circus. At one time he wrote indignantly to *Time* magazine about a woman whose picture they had published under the caption of 'Uglies.' He explained that, previously a vigorous and good-looking woman, she had become the victim of acromegaly and had accepted the offer of Mr. Ringling's agents to pose as 'the ugliest woman in the world' to support her four children, but she 'suffers from intolerable headaches, has become nearly blind, and permits herself to be laughed at and heckled by an unfeeling people. I do not like to feel that *Time* can be frivolous over the tragedies of disease.' "[4]

On a visit to London, he convinced the curator of the Hunterian Museum at the Royal College of Surgeons to allow him to examine the skull of the famous 8ft 2in Irish giant, Charles Byrne. Desirous of his skeleton and much against Byrne's strenuous objections, John Hunter, the great surgical experimentalist, had pursued him to the grave in 1782. Paying an unheard of sum of £100 for the body, he had prepared and mounted the skeleton, which became a long-term public attraction. Cushing confirmed that the man had had a pituitary tumor by the abnormal size of the sella turcica in his skull, the cup-shaped bony depression that cradles and protects the gland.

His lectures and publications on the subject, with careful reference to the other workers interested in the subject, led to his most highly regarded book, *The Pituitary Body and its Disorders*[5] The data were based on 47 of his patients who had had their pituitaries removed via a trans-sphenoidal approach through the nostrils, an approach that he came to prefer to entering the skull directly. He carefully referenced the other workers in the field in the text, primarily those in France and Germany. Published in 1912, the year he moved to the Brigham, the author was identified as "Moseley Professor-Elect of the Peter Bent *Bingham* Hospital."[6]

Every facet of surgery and patient management had to be perfect for the new professor. He refused to accept residents into his program

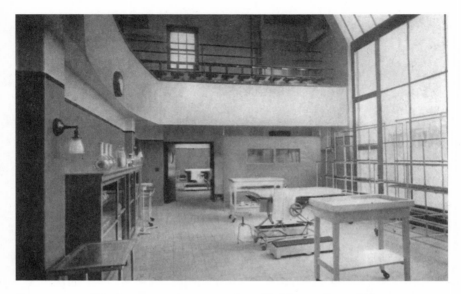

FIGURE 3.1   The large operating room where Cushing performed his
neurosurgical operations.

who were left-handed or married. Intolerant of shortcuts, the many
hours he took to complete his operative procedures were unimportant
if the patient might benefit. In addition to his work on brain tumors,
vascular anomalies, and other central nervous system disorders, he performed fifteen to twenty-five operations on pituitary tumors each year
during his early tenure at the Brigham. His concern with technical
artistry caused him repeatedly to refine existing methods and tools of
surgery to handle the friable and vascular tissues of the brain. Some of
his innovations have become standard in neurosurgery. He initiated
the use of small metal clips to occlude arterial bleeders too deep to tie.
For venous bleeding, he devised the cotton pledget with black silk
markers attached. Alternatively, he placed bits of muscle or blood clots
on the site of bleeding, a precursor of the fibrin foam employed for
homeostasis that one of his trainees, Franc Ingraham, introduced during World War II.

Cushing first tested an electrosurgical unit in the operating room
in 1926, a machine developed by William T. Bovie, a physicist working at an adjacent hospital. This novel device could open tissue by high
frequency interceptive oscillating current and coagulate small vessels

with continuous amplitude current. A former resident described his introduction to the apparatus at a medical meeting the year before. "[We] were watching a demonstration of the use of the dessicating and cutting diathermy machine on a big block of beef. Dr. Cushing came along, stopped to speak to us and in a purely jocular fashion, one of us said 'here is something that you ought to use on the brain!' not that we had any idea that it was applicable there, but I think with the mischievous purpose of stirring Cushing up at the thought of employing such a gross and disgusting procedure as was evidenced in the demonstration. He seemed rather thoughtful. He apparently returned to Boston, and established contact with Bovie."[7]

The first patient on whom he used the apparatus was a 64-year-old man with a highly vascular tumor of the skull that he had tried, unsuccessfully, to excise three days before. Bovie brought his machine to the operating room for a second attempt. Cushing's operative notes

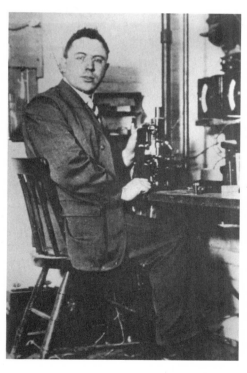

FIGURE 3.2   William T. Bovie (*Ann Plastic Surg* 1979, 2:135).

describe the less than auspicious circumstances: "This operation was a perfect circus. I had persuaded Dr. Bovie to bring his diathermy apparatus over here to let me see what I could do with his cutting loop. This had necessitated re-electrifying the operating room. [An assistant] appeared with four or five coughing Frenchmen with colds in their head. The student who was acting as a possible [blood donor] fainted and fell off the seat. In spite of all this and more, things went surprisingly well. Then with Dr. Bovie's help I proceeded to take off most satisfactorily the remaining portion of tumor with practically none of the bleeding which was occasioned in the preceding operation. The loop acted perfectly and blood spilling was almost completely stopped."[8]

But the machine did not always function smoothly. "On certain occasions in the course of prolonged operations, the body became so heavily charged that the anesthetist on accidentally touching the patient's face could well get a spark which might cause [an] explosion under the hood. Once this occurred, a case in which a small opening had been made into the frontal sinus in the course of a transfrontal osteoplastic operation. This led to a direct communication between the respiratory passages and the field of operation; and suddenly the ether vapor was sparked and went off in a blue flame, fortunately without any injurious effects. Other difficulties experienced at the outset were due to the fact that epileptiform attacks were occasionally produced when the electrode was used to check bleeding from the surface of the dura. Once the operator [Cushing] received a shock which passed through the metal retractor to his arm and out by the wire from his headlight which was unpleasant to say the least." Despite these initial vicissitudes, however, the Bovie cautery and its refinements have become critical components of operating rooms throughout the world.

His meticulous technique and remarkably low infection rate of 0.3% in a pre-antibiotic age reduced patient risk substantially. Indeed, the mortality rate of his operations, reported in 1915, was 8.4%, compared to that of other leading neurosurgeons at the time whose results varied between 38% and 50%.[9] Carl Walter, a surgical expert in hospital epidemiology and hygiene and member of the department, later expanded on this theme. "Neurosurgeons still envy Harvey Cushing, his amazing freedom from sepsis. There is no mystery about it, the Peter Bent Brigham Hospital was extraordinarily well ventilated. The hospital was uncrowded; the high ceilings and deployment of patients assured great cubage per occupant. Visitors were almost banished; the

employee-patient ratio was only 1.6:1. Bedding was disinfected immediately upon discharge. Because of almost total lack of lavatories,
sponges wet with ethanol were dispensed ritualistically to permit disinfection of the hands after every patient contact. The Moseley Professor of Surgery joined administrative white glove rounds frequently
enough to assure immaculate housekeeping.

"Preparation of the operative site was elaborate. A doctor was
assigned to shave the area and to scrub it clean with a soft brush. After
anesthetization the operative site was scrubbed with eight changes of
sponges, alternatively saturated with ethanol and bichloride of mercury. Wet gloves were worn routinely. Surgeons' hands could be identified by the mercury-stained nails. Surgery was done in an
environment purged of bacteria by twenty changes of air per hour.
The operating room floor was kept moist with a phenolic germicide by
repeated and enthusiastic mopping by Adolph Watzka."[10]

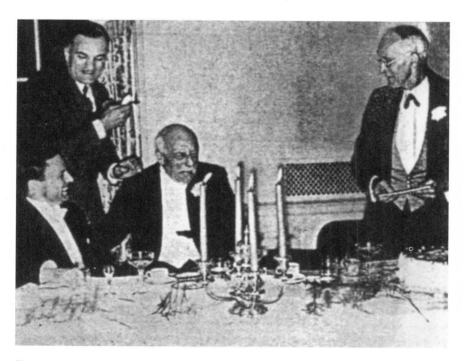

FIGURE 3.3   Adolph Watzka wiping Dr. Krebs's brow during Cushing's 70th
birthday celebration. From Fulton JF, *Harvey Cushing: A Biography* (Oxford:
Blackwell Scientific Publications, Ltd., 1946), 692.

Watzka attended Cushing in many capacities. and continued as operating room orderly until his death in 1956. Virtually indispensable for Cushing, he arranging his surgical headlight, cared for his patients in the operating room, and mopped his brow on hot days. Indeed, to distinguish him from the Brigham interns, the professor made him wear special trousers with blue and white stripes. Adolph was an obvious presence at the opening dinner of the Harvey Cushing Society on April 8, 1939, organized to coincide with Cushing's seventieth birthday. A notable moment occurred when he wiped the beads of perspiration from the bald head of the principal speaker at the beginning of his remarks.

Francis Moore later eulogized this highly visible figure. "Signing up as a hospital orderly he soon showed his skill in mechanical things, his extraordinary devotion to work, and his ability to solve difficult problems in the operative handling of patients. He was a big, heavy-boned, homely man who with great strength achieved complete gentleness, telling the patient exactly what to do to avoid pain or discomfort and with a comforting word. No move was wasted, nothing was done which was unnecessary. It was remarkable to see [him] take hold of a patient, adjust the table or carry out other steps with no face mask. Adolph felt that a face mask limited the freedom of his breathing and that it was unnecessary if he was careful. [He] made a humble chore into a fine profession, and in so doing taught an important lesson to hundreds of young doctors."[11]

Cushing's clinical activity continued unabated throughout his life. His restless intellect and far-ranging scholarship matched his enormous surgical output. This, in turn, allowed him to collect, document, record, and analyze a spectrum of neuroendocrine diseases and other central nervous system disorders. He carefully kept in contact with his patients, often for many years, compiling much follow-up data. His contributions to the medical literature were legion. A talented artist, he illustrated many of his operative notes and papers with detailed drawings of brain lesions. The author of innumerable lectures and essays on a multiplicity of topics, he summarized his surgical philosophy in an address at the University of Liverpool. "Intracranial surgery from a technical standpoint is unlike all other forms of surgery in that the delicate structures involved cannot be handled with a sponge and clamp and ligature as can the tissues of the body with which the surgeon is more familiar. It is far easier to do harm than good by the rough and

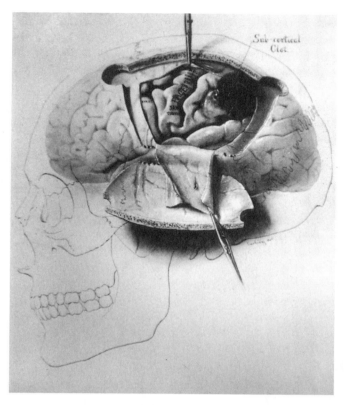

FIGURE 3.4   Cushing's drawing of one of his craniotomy cases, showing a subdural clot. From Thomson EH, *Harvey Cushing: Surgeon, Author, Artist* (New York:
Neale Watson Academic Publications, Inc., 1981), 47.

rapid operative methods so commonly employed. Difficult though it
may often be, the craniotomy itself is the least important element in
the operation. Earlier diagnoses and more prompt interference, a
wider experience in overcoming the technical difficulties of these cases,
coupled with the courage to work slowly and painstakingly, these
things will lead to increasingly better results in this responsible work,
the success of which depends so greatly upon detail, patience and the
expenditure of time."[12]

The single-minded intensity of the new appointee often made him
irascible and perverse to those around him. Indeed, there were mutter-
ings of disapprobation amongst many of his former Boston colleagues

when word came that he had been named to the Brigham position. His complete control over his emotions was illustrated by an instance in 1926 when, following removal of a spinal cord tumor from a young woman, he asked his startled resident to close the dura and then the incision. This departure from the unswerving routine was later explained by the fact that William, Cushing's oldest son and a student at Yale, had been killed that morning in an automobile accident.[13] Although a driving disciplinarian and taskmaster, he engendered intense loyalty amongst his staff and trainees. But even such an energetic and indefatigable worker as Hugh Cairns, later to become the Regius Professor of Surgery at Oxford, noted that his prior experiences as a junior medical officer at Gallipoli in World War I were "nothing compared to the physical stress of a year as Cushing's neurological resident."[14]

At the same time, his legendary charm allowed him to accrue a wide and international circle of friends. Homans describes another telling incident: "Like many other intense persons, Cushing could relax in a delightful way. One evening a young British surgeon who was visiting him suggested that they go to the circus. They did so and enjoyed themselves very well, but at the end of the show, Cushing was not quite satisfied. He suggested that they should look up some of the performers and see what they were like. So off the two went, arm in arm. The circus was packing up, preparing to entrain for another city, and so the investigators ended their search in a freight yard in the car of the tattooed lady. Cushing had no particular knowledge of tattooed ladies in particular, but was so charming and so sympathetic that the very interesting and sensitive woman gave them tea, and told them the touching story of her life. It was like Cushing that, when he did embark on a venture of this sort, his intellectual curiosity should continue active, with results impossible to foresee. It was another of his attractive qualities that he should remember in detail and relate with gusto those experiences and incidents which appealed to his imagination and whimsical sense of humor."[15]

The comments of a former student on the influence of the man are also illuminating: "I heard Dr. Cushing lecture just once to us first year medical students in 1932 when he was on the point of retiring. I remember the imperious way in which he sent the Anatomy Professor, who gave him a flowery introduction, to get a towel to clean off his valuable hands after some chalk had gotten on them from an illustration that he drew on the blackboard. But I also got to know Dr. Cushing through some of the Brigham records which impressed me enormously with his total honesty and thoroughness. One of his operative notes described his partial removal of a bloody meningioma in which he said that he had gone at it all wrong and would do a better job next time in similar circumstances. In another old volume of bound records I found a follow-up note on a patient from whom he had removed a chromophobe adenoma. His resident had written that the patient was much improved in a number of particulars, but Dr. Cushing's note cancelled all that since he said there is no apparent improvement in any way! In my own way I have tried to follow that example of rugged honesty in appraising one's own results, and in that way I suppose that Dr. Cushing left his influence on me without ever having had any personal contact."[16]

AS HEAD OF AN ACTIVE DEPARTMENT, Cushing was forced to deal with a variety of difficult administrative questions. Although he limited increasingly his practice to neurosurgical cases, his enduring interest in general surgical problems that was whetted during his long years with Halsted, continued to intrigue him. Indeed, he remained ambivalent about specialization throughout much of his career, feeling that too many patients with similar disorders such as those with neurologic abnormalities would unbalance the small department. Thus, he insisted that his faculty and trainees cultivate a broad surgical practice and become proficient in a wide range of operations before concentrating on a particular subject or area of the body. On occasion he described neurosurgery as a specialty unto itself. At other times, he emphasized the necessity that it remain under general surgery with its variety of techniques, physiologies and nuances in patient care. His interest in all aspects of the discipline of surgery, combined with his initial failure to be elected to the prestigious American Surgical Association, prompted him to suggest to a few colleagues that they form the Society of Clinical Surgery, to visit each other's clinics and learn what advances they had made in surgical care.

He strongly promoted teaching. With other members of his staff he initiated Saturday morning clinics for the first-year medical students, introducing a comprehensive array of patients and correlating their histories and physical findings with the particular diseases under study at the time. In addition, he strengthened overall surgical educa-

tion by insisting on fewer hours of didactic lectures and more emphasis on bedside instruction. He was vociferously critical of what he considered the rarified attitude of the preclinical instructors at the medical
school who reputedly felt that any reference to the clinical applicability of their material was beneath them. While he lauded the contributions of full-time laboratory investigators to the advancement of
science, he believed that their lack of experience with the ill precluded
proper teaching of medical students. "Here we are struggling to preserve a race of pure preclinical scientists who are unable to reproduce
their species unless we incubate them. I begin to think they waste an
immense amount of the students' time and it would be better if the students began their first two years with clinical work and supplemented
it with such laboratory exercises as their clinical work indicated the
necessity of. I think in this way you will probably get more men interested in science than we do now."[17]

For many years he had held mixed opinions about the impact of the
full-time faculty system on clinical departments. Throughout the history of American medical education, beginning with the founding of
the first medical school in Philadelphia, practitioners whose primary
concerns centered around their private patients carried out clinical
teaching on an ad hoc basis. Only a decade before Cushing left for
Boston, those at Johns Hopkins with the encouragement of and funding from the Rockefeller Foundation initiated a new plan in which the
faculty would be under contract with the university and receive a salary
from funds paid directly to the institution by the patients.

This was a distinct departure from long-established habits of fee
for service. But when the Foundation offered Harvard a similar
arrangement to convert its existing program to the full-time system,
faculty opposition rose high. While Cushing himself disagreed with
several aspects of the proposal, he did feel that the Hopkins system was
more effective than the more laissez-faire, private practice arrangement of the MGH and comparable hospitals of the time, particularly in
providing time for research and increased interaction between the students, the residents, and their teachers. The arrangement at the
Brigham finally became one in which the chiefs of clinical services
would receive a base institutional salary but were allowed a reasonable
amount of private practice using a few beds that the hospital had set
aside for the purpose.

It should be noted that even as Cushing and the Brigham trustees were formulating their financial arrangements for the faculty, the full-time plan had been generating considerable heat, first at Hopkins where it started and later at other university-based medical institutions around the country that had also instituted the arrangement. Halsted and several of his professorial colleagues welcomed the overtures (and money) of the Rockefellers. Osler, with a large private practice in Baltimore, did not. Indeed, he fought hard against such a scheme, fearing "that full time clinicians would be cut off from their patients, and express[ing] the opinion that such a move would shrink them into the dimensions of the laboratory, away from the glories of bedside teaching, resulting in a faculty of 'Halsteds—a very good thing for science but a bad thing for the profession.' He felt it would lead to 'the production of a set of clinical prigs whose only human interest would be research.' "[18] Indeed, Osler's successor as Chair of Medicine, having first welcomed the idea, reconsidered and resigned his position rather than accept the proposed salary.

Cushing summarized his conflicting feelings on the subject in his 1924 *Annual Report*. "A more rigid form of full-time service has been adopted in a few other institutions, primarily at the Johns Hopkins. Larger salaries were given but the incumbents were supposed to be protected against the temptations of having private work interfere too greatly with their hospital duties by having the institution charge and collect the professional fees from private patients. These fees were to be wholly or in part turned back to the department concerned. With either system, abuses may occur. A university hospital having under contract a full paid surgeon and at the same time a private pavilion whose occupants are charged fees, may bring unjustifiable pressure upon him to attend patients and to operate for conditions in which he may happen to be academically uninterested; for he is supposedly a teacher and investigator. On the other hand, a hospital attendant who at the same time holds an academic post may become so engrossed in his personal affairs that he neglects his hospital and academic duties."[19]

The head of the Brigham Board of Trustees emphasized the success of this and other administrative refinements at the twenty-fifth anniversary of the hospital. "The Brigham was the first hospital in America to introduce the modified full-time program for professional staff, an idea which has subsequently spread throughout the nation, and

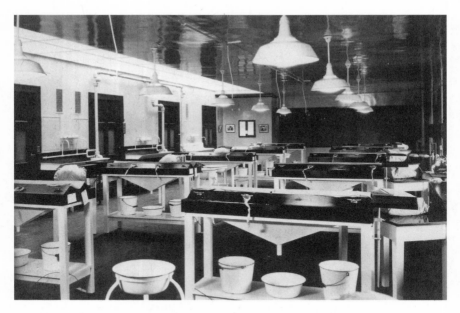

FIGURE 3.5   The Surgical Research Laboratory at Harvard Medical School.

to provide all day out-patient service. It pioneered in establishing a type of resident service, which, by adding to the young house officer a more mature resident group, provided sounder training for the junior medical staff and better continuous service for the patients. Under the genius of its first chief surgeon, Harvey Cushing, and its first chief physician, Henry A. Christian, the hospital developed acknowledged leadership in the care of the sick, the investigations of clinical disorders, and the training of the doctors of the future.[20]

WHILE THE OPERATING ROOM SERVED as a laboratory for Cushing throughout much of his career, he continuously emphasized his enduring belief in the value of an experimental approach to the solution of clinical puzzles carried out in an animal laboratory physically separated from the hospital, by insisting on space in the medical school for a surgical laboratory. As the unfinished hospital was not able to admit patients for a year after his arrival, he and the several resourceful and experienced research colleagues who followed him from the Old Hunterian Laboratory at Hopkins to the Surgical Research Laboratory at Harvard immediately set to work. Lewis Weed, later professor of

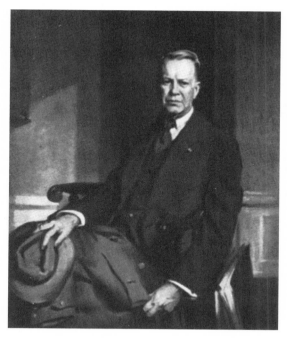

FIGURE 3.6   Lewis Weed, Cushing's first research fellow at Harvard.

anatomy at Hopkins, expanded his seminal observations on the circulation of the cerebrospinal fluid. In a series of papers that comprised virtually an entire issue of the *Journal of Medical Research*, Weed reviewed
the theories of drainage and analyzed existing methods of investigation.
The work has remained a highly publicized and lasting series of classic
experiments. Emile Goetsch, to become professor and chairman of
surgery at Long Island Medical College, continued to examine the puta-
tive role of the pituitary in hibernation, a subject that has come back
recently into vogue. He then devised the "adrenaline test" for patients
with hyperthyroidism. With Conrad Jacobson, soon to enter the surgical residency, Cushing investigated the relationship between the pituitary gland and carbohydrate metabolism. The results of this study led
to a later collaboration with his medical school classmate, the diabetol-
ogist, Elliott Joslin, on the high incidence of diabetes in acromegalic
patients. At the same time, the professor and Clifford Walker, another
young research fellow, worked out the visual field disturbances in
patients with pituitary tumors that pressed on the optic nerves.

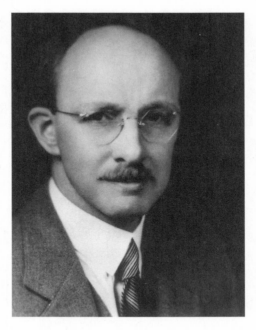

Figure 3.7   Emil Holman as Chief Resident, 1924.

Within a few years, Emil Holman while chief resident completed an extensive and clinically applicable series of experiments on arteriovenous fistula, a long-standing subject of interest to surgeons. Anatomist William Hunter (John's brother) had first described a direct communication between an artery and a vein in 1761. More than a century later, a Georgia surgeon noted enlargement of the heart of a patient who had developed a fistulous aneurysm of his femoral vessels after a gunshot wound. "The most mysterious phenomenon connected with the case was slowing of the heart's beat when compression of the common femoral was employed."[21] Others commented on its occurrence but were unable to explain it. Holman surgically anastomosed major arteries and veins in dogs and reported in a series of important papers that the loudness of the murmur heard over the vessels depended on fistula size and free return of blood to the heart.[22] Large fistulae produced circulatory insufficiency with a rapid pulse rate and decline in blood pressure. The heart compensated by increasing in size. These changes, however, reverted to normal on closing the connection.

By happenstance, one of Cushing's patients, Charles Mundi, provided Holman with the chance to confirm his experimental observations.[23] This 42-year-old man had developed progressive paraplegia associated with an arteriovenous aneurysm from a gunshot wound of the groin sustained 25 years previously. A thrill was felt. The aorta and iliac artery were greatly enlarged. After Homans closed the fistula, blood pressure and pulse rate normalized and the enlarged heart decreased in size. The observations of this young surgical investigator about this phenomenon and its physiology have never been improved upon.

The productivity of these research workers and the quality of their experimental work quickly substantiated to those remaining skeptics the benefits and importance of a well-organized and manned surgical laboratory with strong ties to a clinical service. Indeed, the rapid success of Cushing's new laboratory contrasted dramatically with its previous precarious existence despite Warren's efforts, with meager funds and no designated director to organize or supervise individual projects. To aid in its support, a fellowship fund was established in 1912 named after Arthur Tracy Cabot, a member of the MGH staff. The fellowship provided the Moseley Professor of Surgery the means to select a likely member of the resident group to spend a year full-time working in and supervising the research laboratory, a strategy he had already established at Hopkins. The experience would teach the incumbent the value of precise experimentation, and encourage meticulous, accurate, and detailed recording of observations. Most importantly, it would allow him an unbroken period of time to concentrate upon a particular problem. This opportunity for independent thinking, thoughtful inquiry, and exploration of a given field freely using their own talents drew many of the chosen young men into productive academic careers.

Cushing soon found that creating a new department with its administrative load, teaching, and increasing clinical responsibilities kept him from the laboratory. However, as he had learned from Halsted, he trained his residents by insisting on close ties between those with clinical responsibilities and those involved in experimental research. Staying in touch with the current projects, he spent much time with his assistants in preparing their manuscripts, carefully detailing the bibliography and illustrations, and encouraging a dramatic style of writing. His support of and accessibility to his young house staff and his love of teaching was obvious. One described such an instance. "A few months into the job, wishing to try my hand at writing, I asked the head of radiology, if he had something that I might work up into a report. When the study [of patients whose carbuncles were treated with x-ray] was completed, I asked Dr. Cushing to read it and comment. On the following Sunday morning he phoned to tell me to meet him at his office at 9:30—a rare event, since he never came to the hospital on Sundays except for emergencies. For an hour and a half he led me through the skills and subtleties of writing a scientific paper, giving special emphasis to the opening sentence and the closing paragraph. I left the office walking on air. To have this busy man, at the height of his career, go to such trouble for a junior house officer made me light-headed."[24]

Cushing's concept of himself as head of the department of surgery at Harvard did not please many in the Harvard administration who felt that neither all branches of surgery should be under the jurisdiction of one man nor that surgical investigations were important. His enthusiasm for deans was never great, declaiming that "they should all be in the cellar and the more prisonlike the quarters, the better."[25] The dean with whom his animosity lasted longest was David Edsall. Moving from a successful career as a clinical investigator to the deanship, Edsall, a highly prominent figure at the time, may have unintentionally grated upon Cushing's sensibilities by assuming a somewhat superior posture toward surgeons who involved themselves in research. The attitude long held by many physicians that surgeons might not really be capable of high intellectual effort may further have inflamed an already discordant relationship between the two. An effective and conscientious administrator, Edsall disagreed with the professor constantly on various matters in general and on the surgical laboratory in particular. Indeed, his research facilities had been a sore point with Cushing since his original appointment and contributed to ongoing misunderstandings.

To accommodate the needs of other departments, those in charge at the medical school forced the laboratory to move to less attractive quarters in 1923.[26] Much against his wishes but on the urging of the dean and various influential members of the administrative board, Cushing agreed on the understanding that the new quarters would be as satisfactory as those they had to vacate. Heated correspondence regarding the move passed between Edsall, Cushing, and the Committee on Space during the three-year period of planning.[27] As the animal quarters also had to be transferred and adequate accommodations were not forthcoming, small, inconvenient, and occasionally insurmountable problems developed. "Recently Dr. Wislocki (Cabot Fellow and eventually Professor of Anatomy at Harvard) kept his deer in the outside space and packed animal food was kept inside. He is now interested in knowing how to obtain space in the animal house to which he feels entitled. What shall I tell him?"[28] Other more subtle difficulties were never resolved. "I do not know precisely the person with whom I should take up the question of dogs barking."[29] Despite continued assurances of a smooth transition, the end result provoked Cushing to fire a testy fusillade at Edsall.

"You will, of course, recall that the Surgical Laboratory with many protests from me and others was moved from its long established quarters to its present quarters. With a good many misgivings, I finally submitted with the understanding that we were to have the entire floor, that our accommodations would be as comparable to those we have recently had as circumstances permitted. I was abroad during the summer then on my return found to my dismay that our supplies had merely been tumbled into the rooms and I even had a great deal of difficulty in getting our predecessors to vacate.

"I have never issued heretofore any complaints or protests though I have always felt it was a very small action on the part of the school to oust us from our quarters and then neglect us after we were moved. I am bringing this whole story to your attention because I trust that you can see your way clear at least to reimbursing the Department for the unexpectedly heavy expenses that they have been called upon to meet in providing for even makeshift arrangements for the care of animals."[30]

Monetary support for the laboratory was a source of chronic difficulty for Cushing, particularly as the facilities were also used to instruct the medical students in surgical technique in dogs. University scholarship funds supported the Cabot Fellows and the hospital and/or the medical school sometimes grudgingly carried the general laboratory deficits. Gifts and philanthropic foundations helped to sustain surgical investigators who donated their time in pursuing specific problems. Indeed, the research budget never increased after 1912 except for a few hundred dollars for office expenses. The annual expenditures for the surgery and pathology laboratories, artists, and photography in the years after World War I totaled over $35,000, the majority of which the professor covered with private funds. By 1923, the situation had become so acute that Cushing could not accommodate those desiring to work. Personal money from appreciative patients and other donors increasingly financed the salaries of the few laboratory technicians, as well as the research projects themselves. Funds from the medical school were rarely forthcoming.

In 1925, pressures building between Cushing and Edsall finally exploded. The dean believed he saw an opportunity to secure an endowment for the surgical laboratory and requested Cushing, with full reasons for his request, to provide a summary of its accomplishments of the past several years accompanied by a rationale for the existence of such a separate laboratory distinct geographically from the hospital. Apparently, Cushing concluded from this request that the Medical School was trying to wrest control of his space. He penned a reply that vented several years of accumulated annoyance and frustration, presaging a theme that was to recur intermittently over the entire 90-year existence of the Surgical Research Laboratory.[31]

"You asked me in your letter if I would at my leisure give you: (1) A statement of the accomplishments during the last few years of the research laboratory; (2) The arguments for the existence of such a separate laboratory. I may well enough answer question (1) by supplying you with the titles of papers published from the laboratory since 1912. It might suffice as an answer to your question (2) to give you a list of the Arthur Tracy Cabot Fellows and the present positions they occupy. Without doubt, the training these men received in the Surgical Laboratory had no little part in the subsequent success they have obtained. In further answer to your second question, I may take it for granted that the members of any major departments in the school—perhaps the Department of Surgery more than any other, need opportunities and encouragement to engage in laboratory investigations. Surgical problems, moreover, are ones which for their solution usually necessitate the use of animals. The surgical laboratory, too, is a place where students should have their first experience in the making and repairing of operative wounds. To my great disappointment this has been made practically impossible in the Harvard Medical School, particularly through lack of funds, partly through the actions of the curriculum committee—in short, for the want of school support. If a referendum were to be put before the students in any school in which a proper course of operative surgery on animals is being given, I venture to say that 90% would regard it as the most valuable practical experience in their entire school course. Furthermore, I may add that within the present day, no candidate for a Chair in Surgery would for a moment be considered eligible by any of our leading schools who had not himself had experience in research and who was thereby at least capable of stimulating others with the quest of knowledge. Conversely, no surgeon of the caliber decided by our leading schools to be head of the Department would for a minute consider accepting a Chair of Surgery unless ample opportunities for laboratory work supported by an ample budget were provided.

"These, then, are some *general reasons* for the continued existence of a 'separate surgical laboratory.' But if you ask for *specific reasons*, I may say that when I accepted a position here at Harvard, the only request I made was for better facilities for the care of animals. I little realized until I came here that it would be necessary to solicit funds from outside sources to meet ordinary running expenses. Had it not been that the A.T. Cabot Fellowship was at my disposal, so that I could put a full-time worker in the laboratory, without the school having to call upon its general funds to pay for such a person, the laboratory ere this would almost certainly have been closed. But this is not all, for the benefit of another department; the laboratory was forced to give up its large library space. Again, by still another department, it was forced to give up its entire quarters and to be moved to much less desirable and commodious ones in another building. We are now asked what is the good of the Surgical Laboratory at all? In fact, no opportunity or encouragement for surgical research exists here in any way comparable to those I enjoyed as an Associate Professor of the Johns Hopkins 12 years ago ... Since my coming here it has been a constant struggle even to keep the laboratory running, far less to use it extensively as a teaching adjunct to the Department.

"I might pursue the answers to these questions much further, but have perhaps said enough. When all emphasis today is laid upon scientific and laboratory work, for anyone to imply that the clinician and perhaps above all the surgeon [whose] energy and time is expended in laborious hours of the operating table, should receive discouragement from the School in regard to the pursuit of knowledge is to me amazing. One might well suggest that the physiologist carry out their researches in the laboratories of the Anatomical Department. If the preclinical departments succeed in driving the clinician out of the school entirely, instead of encouraging him to work there, it will be one more source of estrangement between those departments which deal with patients and those which do not."[32]

In response to these and other missives hurled between their offices, the Surgeon-in-Chief at the Brigham and the Dean at Harvard Medical School made a few attempts to assuage the situation. "Now as for my testy note—which so riled you that you forwarded it to the President [of Harvard]. I think both of us have had too much on our shoulders the week before, and I am glad that you have at least gotten away for a vacation."[33] Poor Edsall! His only recourse was to drop occasional and plaintive comments to President Lowell: "Dr. Cushing, as you know, is one of the most difficult of the men in the group to deal with and is constantly looking for slights and constantly tending to stir up a sense of injustice. I do not think that he does any particular harm in this way. Dr. Cushing's brilliancy and accomplishments and his value in the school are beyond question."[34]

CUSHING'S SURGICAL STAFF carried much of the burden of the department during his enduring involvement in the events of World War I. As his international contacts and interests made him particularly aware of the strong German threat in Europe, he found himself increasingly at odds with the isolationist temper of the United States in the years preceding the conflict. With the outbreak of hostilities American residents in Paris organized a military hospital and motor ambulance core to be staffed in rotation by volunteer physicians and nurses from a few important university hospitals. George Crile organized a unit from his department at Western Reserve; Cushing and a colleague from the MGH established a Harvard unit. A group from the University of Pennsylvania superceded them in turn. When Cushing and his contingent arrived in France in April 1915, the war had been ongoing for eight months and the wounded had begun to accumulate in large numbers. His initial reactions were overwhelming.

"It is difficult to say just what are one's most vivid impressions: The amazing patience of the seriously wounded, some of them hanging on for months; the dreadful deformities (not so much in the way of amputations, but broken jaws and twisted, scarred faces); the tedious healing of the infected wounds, with discharging sinuses, tubes, irrigations, and repeated dressings—so much so that grafting and painful fractures are simply abandoned to wait for wounds to heal, which they don't do;

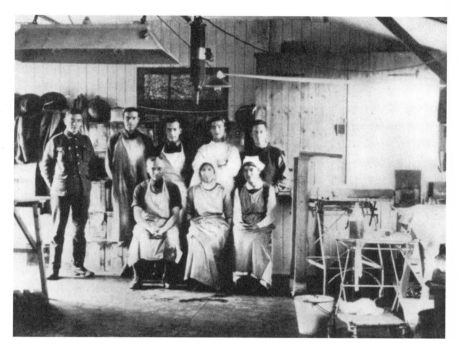

FIGURE 3.8   Cushing and his operating team at Boulogne, 1917. From Cushing H, *From a Surgeon's Journal* (Boston: Little, Brown, and Co., 1936), 254.

the risks under apparently favorable circumstances of attempting clean operations, most of which seem to have broken down."[35]

Operating, observing, visiting, inspecting, and recording it all, Cushing became saturated by his experience at the Front before returning to Boston. His subsequent attempts to produce a Base Hospital were generally unsuccessful until the declaration of war by President Wilson in April 1917, when the entire Harvard unit was quickly ordered to mobilize for France; Crile's unit was the only other in the country even approximately ready. Cushing rapidly organized and shepherded Base Hospital Number 5 onto the *S. S. Saxonia* which landed in France at the end of May 1917.

The situation that he and his group faced was difficult. "A shockingly dirty, unkempt camp" with vast numbers of the wounded requiring care, far worse than he had seen two years before. The numbers were staggering. Those already there told him that 8,000 patients had passed through the Base Hospital in a few weeks; he later recorded 499 patients seen in 27 hours, evacuating four patients a minute.[36] The pace was uncontrolled, the pressures unrelenting. "Operating from 8:30 a.m. one day until 2:00 a.m. the next, standing in a pair of rubber boots and periodically full of tea as a stimulant, is not healthy. It is an awful business, probably the worst possible training at surgery for a young man, and ruinous for carefully acquired techniques of an old- ster." The conditions in the trenches were frightful, with often-con- tinuous rain liquefying the mud. Vast numbers of soldiers died of infection and exposure. More died from their wounds. "A lot of wounded men must have drowned in the mud. Urgent operations on more rotting men. In the early afternoon a large batch of wounded were unexpectedly brought in—mostly heads—men who have been lying out for four days in craters in the rain, without food."[37] Again: "One of the trains dumped about 500 badly wounded men, and left them lying between the tracks in the rain, with no cover whatsoever. One English officer who had been six days thus in transport, with a musket for a splint tied to a compound fracture of the femur, no dress-

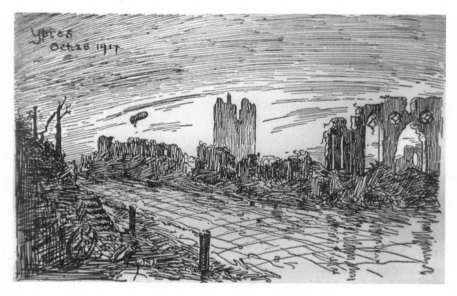

FIGURE 3.9   Cushing's drawing of the desolation of Ypres, 1917. From Cushing H, *From a Surgeon's Journal*, 245.

ing whatsoever, almost no food or drink; he was in delirium when he arrived. Fortunately, the wounded were young and in the pink of physical condition; few would otherwise have pulled through."[38]

Musing on the cessation of hostilities, his feelings seemed to predict too clearly events to come throughout much of the remaining century. "Too tired, squalid and uncomfortable to talk to each other, we scarcely needed to do so while familiar shibboleths resound in our ears—that this was to be the war to end all wars, and that the world from now on will be made safe for democracy. We wonder."[39]

In addition to his huge surgical workload, traveling, and chronicling his experiences at the Front, he kept extensive individual patient records of the thousands of men on whom he had operated, a record constituting the only series of the neurologically wounded reported in detail from the War. In an article published in 1919, he described 119 such patients.[40] Remarkably, Hugh Cairns produced a follow-up report of the same individuals in 1942.[41] Cushing even found time to cultivate friendships with Sir Almroth Wright of Saint Mary's Hospital in London, largely responsible for immunizing the entire British Expeditionary Force against typhoid, and Alexis Carrel who with English chemist Henry Dakin tested and perfected a series of antiseptic solutions for use in war wounds. His articles on the management of cranial injuries sustained in war and the opportunity to study neurophysiological events following selective injury had enormous influence on later neurosurgical thinking, particularly during World War II[42] From his diaries, which filled nine bound volumes, he published in 1936 to general acclaim his observations and sensations in a single volume, *From a Surgeon's Journal.*[43]

THE PROFESSOR'S EFFICIENT USE of time allowed him the opportunity not only to travel widely but to enhance his growing bibliophilic association with Sir William Osler in Oxford.[44] Despite his alleged early aversion to the printed word both in the extensive family library in Cleveland and during his undergraduate years, Osler and his other supporters in Baltimore kindled his interest in books into a lifelong passion. His growing collection also encouraged him to take multiple trips to England after Osler had moved there, his visits often turning into a joint bibliophilic and antiquarian feast. Initially interested in the history of anatomic illustration, particularly the works of Vesalius, he later expanded his collection into the history of surgery, and eventually

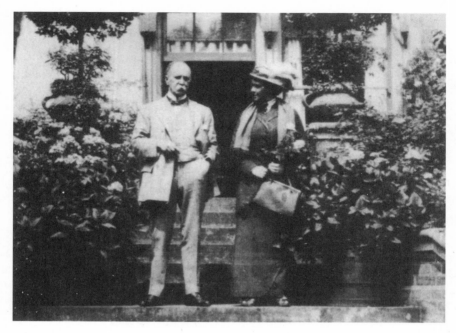

FIGURE 3.10   Sir William and Lady Osler at their house in Oxford. From Wagner FB, *The Twilight Years of Lady Osler: Letters of a Doctor's Wife* (Canton, MA: Science History Publications, USA, 1985), 14.

the history of medicine in general. He never catalogued his books. Undertaking this task only after his death, his biographer, John Fulton, found 15,000 volumes of astonishing quality.[45] Indeed, one of his most enduring legacies was his collection of medical books and incunabula which became the basis of a great medical historical library at Yale.

His friendship with William Osler was one of the most fulfilling of his life. Visiting Oxford after his first tour in France in 1915, he received "a warm greeting and a quiet family dinner after which delightful glimpses of Sir William's wonderful collection of books and manuscripts. Also talk of Revere's [Osler's only son] growing interest in bibliography and the recent hoax which he, with his friend played on his father—the fictitious sale of his valuable library in the hands of a hermit book collector in Norwich."[46]

While in France again two years later, Cushing received word that Revere Osler, now in the Army, had been seriously wounded. Arriving on the scene earlier, Crile had tried unsuccessfully to repair the massive intra-abdominal injuries. Cushing later reported somberly: "We saw him buried in the early morning. A soggy Flanders field, an overcast windy day—the long rows of simple wooden crosses—the new ditches half full of water, the boy wrapped in an Army blanket and covered by a weather worn union jack, carried on the shoulders of four slipping stretcher bearers."[47] Much correspondence about this tragedy flew between Cushing in France and Osler in Oxford. While his presence certainly helped, his mentor and friend never recovered from the loss. Osler died two years later.

In 1920, Lady Osler requested Cushing to write Sir William's biography. As Osler had acted as confidant and father figure to him for two decades, as well as germinating and fostering his antiquarian interests, the opportunity could not be denied. Taking time off from his departmental duties to work in Oxford, he submitted a manuscript of almost one million words to the Oxford University Press in 1924. At their insistence, he cut this to about a third the length. A remarkable and enthusiastic reception followed publication of *The Life of Sir William Osler*, culminating in the Pulitzer Prize for Biography in

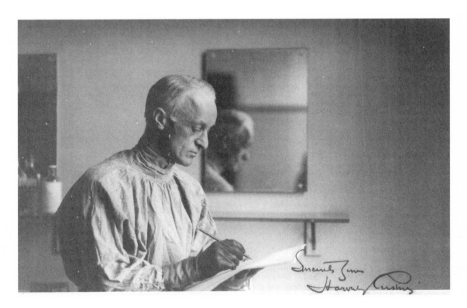

FIGURE 3.11   Cushing in the later period of his career.

1926.[48] The painstaking detail of the book mirrored Cushing himself. However, the complete absence of his name in the text (indeed, going to some lengths to avoid its use) was hardly typical of the man in whom excessive modesty was less than an obvious trait.

Even during this later period of his career, his clinical workload at the Brigham and production of papers and reports remained undiminished. Following his example, several of his pupils and colleagues began to compile and publish their own figures on surgical mortality for tumors of the brain. These, combined with the ongoing productivity of Homans, Cheever and others, consistently increased the national and international academic profile of his small department.

CHAPTER 4

THE ORIGINAL
SURGICAL STAFF

MANY TEACHING HOSPITALS in North America and Western Europe have excelled through their consistent contributions to scientific and clinical knowledge. A specific subject of interest may endure for many years through the work of succeeding generations of faculty. Not infrequently, a single individual within an academic department has opened, broadened, or refined a field not only by his or her original ideas but by stimulating the creativity of collaborators and trainees through drive, enthusiasm, or example. The resultant area of productivity, once established, may lead to new questions, trigger new avenues of investigation, and engender new interests and applications. This theme has been a constant one throughout the history of the Brigham.

What was there about Cushing that made him pre-eminent as a surgical leader and one who set a tone of sustained achievement by members of his department? With a few others, he developed an entirely new specialty. Although cosmopolitan and international in scope and with a well-developed sense of inquiry into a broad array of both medical and non-medical topics, he took infinite time and trouble to ensure the comfort of each of his patients. In addition to his vaunted expertise in endocrine diseases, neurophysiology, brain tumors, and other central nervous system disorders, his professional interests were protean and included investigations into cardiac surgery, local anesthesia, veterinary diseases, and patient monitoring in the operating room. His clinical recall was complete as was his ability to cut through less critical facts and data to understand the larger order of things. This intuitive approach toward human biology motivated him to develop and apply concepts ahead of those that ultimately became accepted as routine. His unremitting energies and industry allowed him to examine, record, and influence many branches of both the sciences and the humanities.

One of his principal attributes was the ability to surround himself with a coterie of able surgical colleagues and disciples who advanced surgery and surgical research substantially. During his tenure at Hopkins and then at the Brigham, he had created an atmosphere so dynamic that talented young men flocked to join him to gain not only the qualities of conscientious patient care and the ability to perform complex surgical manipulations deftly and successfully, but the curiosity to question or enhance existing scientific dogma. This enduring spirit drove many of them to become creative and imaginative figures in their chosen fields. The reputation Cushing had gained on his move to the Brigham continued to attract highly qualified individuals. John Homans and David Cheever formed the nucleus of his new clinical faculty.

JOHN HOMANS (1877–1954) was the fourth of his family to practice medicine in Boston. After attending Harvard College and Harvard Medical School, he interned at the MGH under Maurice Richardson, the most prominent surgeon in the city. Richardson "was sensitive to the fact that the best scientific work of the day was being done elsewhere; that Boston had become a medical backwater, [and emphasized] the damage wrought by institutional conservatism."[1] In reaction, he arranged that his protégé join Cushing at the Old Hunterian Laboratory to examine the endocrine function of the pituitary and the pancreas. "I write on behalf of my assistant, John Homans. I suggested to him that the very best thing he could do would be to go to Baltimore and do some work under your direction. I look upon him as one of the brightest assistants that I have ever had. I feel that my men, although they make splendid practitioners of surgery, fail to gain any inspiration toward so-called research work. Of course we are seeking all the time—and hoping that we shall find knowledge in the fields of practical surgery; but it seems that the coming generation needs a broader field in which to work, that the men should be more than clinical observers. It is a good thing to have a very broad foundation upon which to base special knowledge and experience. I feel, too, that we get to be very narrow in Boston."[2] Following additional training in London with the physiologist Ernest H. Starling, Homans returned to

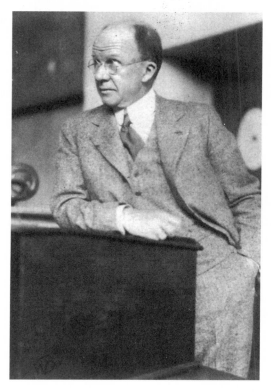

Figure 4.1   John Homans at the podium, 1929 (*J Vasc Surg* 1996, 23:1077).

Boston at Cushing's invitation in 1912. He remained on the Brigham surgical staff throughout the bulk of his surgical career.

In the tradition of competent and careful surgeons who spend much time with their patients, Homans believed and taught that reason and the five senses were of more use in examining, probing, and diagnosing than laboratory technology and erudite physiology. Unmoved by existing dogma, his approach to disease was straightforward. He decried the division between medical disciplines, noting that the surgeon must no longer be a barber or craftsman, but an internist as well. A highly visible and colorful character of volatile temperament and with a vocabulary occasionally replete with uninhibited sobriquets and epithets, he influenced generations of medical students and house staff in the care of the surgically ill. He is remembered as a balding man with a rolling gait, sparkling eyes, a rollicking wit and a contagious laugh. Greatly enjoying his own jokes, he wrinkled up his face into a mischievous expression as he peered at his colleagues to see if they shared in the humor of the occasion. He often spoke loudly, even about delicate matters, believing that clarity should supercede subtlety. His bright, facile mind not infrequently caused his words to stumble out over each other in the form of a rapid lisp. He was frank with his patients, admitting "I am not all sure that I did the right operation. We will have to wait and see!"[3]

Years later, Chilton Crane, a long-term member of the Brigham staff, recalled "Professor John Homans, distinguished laboratory researcher, medical writer and historian, general surgeon especially interested in the venous and lymphatic circulations. Dr. Homans was an original thinker, with a warm and friendly personality, a puckish, bubbling, chuckling sense of humor, and with endless numbers of admiring patients. He bobs down the corridor of private ward A Main on his cane to find not a single nurse in sight. Without an instant's hesitation, he would sit at the nurses' desk, grab the tall black telephone, ring the operator, at the front of the hospital and say: 'Please call A Main' and hang up. The telephone would ring furiously and three nurses would rush out of different rooms. He'd say: 'Thank you, Operator, that's all' and hang up. Then he'd turn to the nearest nurse, and say: 'Miss, would you take me to see Mrs. Fritz in room 9?' He would flash a glance of minor triumph at any observer.

"He was secretly rebellious of many operating room sterility precautions. He regarded them as rigid guidelines for students, not firm rules for experienced surgeons. After scrubbing hands and forearms for two minutes, not five, instead of shutting off the long armed faucet handles with his elbows, he would give a mischievous look at his assistant scrubbing beside him, reach up and quickly shut off the faucets with his freshly scrubbed hands. He knew there were many more bacteria on the washed legs of his varicose vein patients than on those faucets."[4] In contrast, his colleague, David Cheever, a more circumspect personality, scrubbed at "a separate, engraved, wall-mounted silver basin, provided by a generous patient. That sight prompted John Homans to comment on the 'saintly hands of some surgeons,' promoting acrimony over their different aseptic techniques" and undoubtedly driving the more rigid Cheever to distraction.

Crane continues: "Many of his patients were old first name friends of his. They so adored him and had such overwhelming faith in him that he liked to mildly shock them in the operating room. While a nurse was holding up a patient's legs by the gloved feet while the resident scrubbed them with Zephiran, Dr. Homans would come in the room to put on his gown. 'Miriam,' he'd say in a loud voice, 'you know, I don't have the faintest idea what operation I'm going to do today.' He'd look over at the resident to get a kick out of his surprise. 'But, John, it will be on my veins, won't it?' 'Of course, that's why we're washing them off so well!' 'Well, John, you go right ahead. You know what's best and I don't.'

"On a personal note (even though I observed all of the above), after I had presented a surgical case at x-ray conference, Dr. Homans came up to me afterwards to say, in his whiney voice, 'Crane, you presented that case very nicely. But, to mix the bitter with the sweet, you must learn to keep your hands out of your pockets.'

"One Saturday morning at a first year anatomy clinic in the operating room with a hundred students peering down from the stands above, Dr. Homans was excising the lymph soaked subcutaneous tissue from the elephantiasic leg of a twenty-one-year-old girl. Richard Warren was first assisting and I was the pup passing instruments. Dr. Warren had already placed all twenty of the snaps the kit called for along the edges of the long incision. As Dr. H kept cutting away and Rich kept reaching out for more hemostats, I began taking them off down by the ankle where he had started and handing them up. Soon brisk bleeding followed this process so I whispered to Rich that the ankle was bleeding. He said quietly: 'Dr. Homans, we're having some bleeding at the lower leg.' Dr. Homans glanced down and said in a loud voice that reverberated through the amphitheater: 'My God! A hemorrhage!' With that he pounced on the leg to make pressure with a mic pad. This sudden, dramatic announcement by the professor, caused the impressionable students to almost fall forward out of their seats with renewed interest in the operation."[4]

Other than his clinical expertise and the critical shepherding of students and young surgeons through their early years, the output of his pen was his greatest contribution. His 1931 *Textbook of Surgery* was a milestone, treasured by generations of medical students. A master at stimulating those about him to involve themselves either in laboratory investigations or in clinical writing, Cushing had blandly suggested that Homans collate and edit the lectures that the surgical staff presented each year to the students into a "Harvard Textbook of Surgery." Persuaded to undertake the project, he found himself receiving material ranging from literary masterpieces, to skeleton notes, to nothing at all. Although the latter category included the professor's own contribution, Cushing's further encouragement convinced his victim to continue in a manner consistent with his peers and the institution sponsoring the project.

For seven years Homans labored until he had created a work of 1,100 pages, styled and reworked completely by himself into a uniform and complete text. It was a vast and often discouraging project. In the end, however, from a collection of diverse, unbalanced, and spotty notes, he created a book that became a flowing and readable series of essays on all aspects of surgery then current.

His humor shines throughout the text. He wrote clearly, interspersing facts with entertaining phrases and using drawings and sketches almost exclusively in lieu of x-rays and photographs. William Shepherd, a pupil of the distinguished Johns Hopkins medical illustrator, Max Brödel, drew the expressive pictures. Again at Cushing's suggestion, the author included a brief but informative historical summary at the beginning of each chapter to catch the attention of the readers. Several of these introductions are classics, including one describing the important but involuntary part that females played in the evolution of surgery. "Woman has been subject to many critical surgical experiments. The earliest trial battles with bacteria were found in midwifery, and the first steps in abdominal surgery were attempting to heal by operative means the great ovarian cysts, which for ages had carried endless disability and suffering. It is now almost impossible to imagine the number of invalids, with swollen abdomens and drawn, pinched faces who were ready, when surgery could [provide] even a fighting chance of relief, to offer themselves for hazardous operations."[5] A mood of misanthropy surfaced, however, when he described lower abdominal pain which "is so far as I know the most baffling symptom known to surgery and occurs as a rule in females of almost unparalleled dreariness." Other flavorful remarks included a discussion on surgical technique. "In surgery, as in every other art, fundamental matters are perennially being discovered, discredited, forgotten, rediscovered and reaffirmed."[6] He began his chapter on the spleen with the comment: "The spleen always seems to have been counted as a sort of deglomming organ. A large spleen encourages laughter; a small one, melancholy."[7]

In his review of the book for the *New England Journal of Medicine*, Cushing praised the author as well as the other faculty members whose lecture notes contributed to its initial stages. He concluded: "Here is a book about surgery to read, the like of which to the writer's knowledge has not been produced in modern times. The Irishism that Osler's *Medicine* was the best existent work written on surgery has often been repeated. It was a book, in other words, that the surgeons could not well be without. But now we have a work on surgery which a physician cannot well be without, for sanely and picturesquely it gives just the sort of information about his colleague's problems and point of view that he needs to have at hand. And so far as concerns the undergraduate student for whom the work is primarily intended, this is a book, like Osler's which is as easy reading as a novel."[8]

A personalized document, the textbook went through six editions, the last published in 1945. It possessed so much of the author's personality and character within it that not surprisingly he could never convince any younger colleague to carry on the work.

While Homans's early scientific writings were concerned with his endocrine experiments and various general surgical topics, the major subject of interest throughout the majority of his career and about which he studied, spoke, and wrote widely, involved the manifestations and complications of diseases of the veins and obstruction of the lymphatics of the lower extremity. His many investigations into causes and effects of the swollen leg established a subject of interest that continued at the Brigham for decades.

He first defined the patterns of venous drainage of the leg and the causes of varicose veins. Normally, blood moves from the saphenous vein to the deep system and eventually to the heart. If a valve in that superficial vein, often at the groin, becomes incompetent, the weight of the column of blood distally causes the vessel below to dilate. Valves further down the leg become incompetent as the channel enlarges. Varicosities develop. If very large, they may erode the skin and form a simple ulcer, usually at the ankle. In contrast, thrombophlebitis, inflammation of the vessel wall with clot formation, may inhibit venous return by obstructing the deep vein. In this circumstance, blood flows to the superficial vessels via incompetent communicating branches. These, in turn, dilate and may leak plasma into the surrounding tissues.

The leg becomes chronically swollen. The overlying skin thickens and becomes inflamed. Extensive ulcers may result. In classifying the various types of leg ulcers, Homans showed that he could cure the simple lesions by stripping the superficial venous channels but that interruption of the large feeder veins from the deep system was necessary to treat the more complex and severe post-phlebitic changes. He later excised and grafted the ulcer.[9]

His studies on the chronically swollen leg also alerted his colleagues to the significance of lymphatic obstruction. Clinical investigators had long known that thrombophlebitis was only one cause of leg swelling, and that lymphatic, but not venous obstruction was responsible for the edematous arms that patients developed after mastectomy for breast cancer.[10] Intrigued by such evidence, Homans began to study the role of lymphatic obstruction in patients with edematous lower extremities.[11] Having classified the common lymphedemas (filarial, surgical, familial, or sporadic), he and his collaborators produced elephantiasis in a series of dogs, noting that the resultant brawny and indurated subcutaneous tissues were susceptible to and aggravated by repeated episodes of acute infection.[12] As in his patients, lymphostasis eventually advanced to fibrosis and scarring, sometimes profoundly deforming the extremity. He treated mild cases effectively with pressure bandages and elevation of the leg at night. Severe cases demanded operative removal of a finite mass of swollen and edematous tissue. The retained skin flaps were laid directly on the muscle beneath. Performed in stages, these operations restored some degree of convenience and cosmesis to seriously afflicted patients.

Homans's later investigations into thromboembolism from deep thrombosis of the lower extremities caused him to recommend prophylactic ligation of the superficial femoral vein. He was the first in the United States to perform portacaval shunts on patients with liver disease and portal hypertension. His important and original contributions culminated in 1939 in a monograph, *Circulatory Diseases of the Extremities.*[13]

Except for two years in the army in Europe during World War I and a sabbatical year at Yale toward the end of his career, Homans spent his entire professional life at the Brigham. Sometimes gruff, often amusing, always individualistic, he was of the group of surgeons who left a legacy of concern for his patients, an inquiring mind, and an unquenched enthusiasm for his specialty. These traits stimulated deeply those whom he taught.

DAVID CHEEVER (1876–1955) was the other member of Cushing's original surgical faculty. Appointed with Homans, he remained at the Brigham throughout his entire career. A Bostonian, he was reserved and formal in temperament.[14] Of scholarly inclinations, one of his favorite pastimes as an undergraduate at Harvard had been to meet informally with his peers and professors to discuss weighty issues and topics of the day. Graduating from Harvard Medical School in 1901, he originally wanted to follow the career of his father, a brilliant ovariotimist, one of Cushing's surgical mentors, and seventh president of the American Surgical Association. Hardworking, God-fearing, and of Puritan stock, the Cheevers were a conservative and high-principled group. Indeed, surgery had been a tradition in the family since an ancestor had served in that capacity during the Revolutionary War.

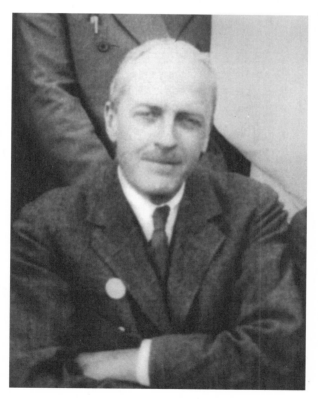

FIGURE 4.2   David Cheever.

Cheever volunteered with the British Expeditionary Forces in France at the outbreak of World War I, eventually heading the surgical arm of the Harvard unit in Boulogne in 1915. After returning to Boston, he acted as surgeon-in-chief during Cushing's war service in France two years later and again during Elliott Cutler's absence during World War II.[15] He described his sentiments about this latter assignment in the 1942 *Annual Report*: "It is for us to give an accounting of our stewardship during this period briefly and without complaint, with our thoughts sympathetically embracing the millions of human beings who have been plunged into grief, sorrow, and unspeakable suffering by the maniacal folly of a few monsters in human form."[16]

He had worked in the department of anatomy at the medical school before beginning his clinical training. With these dual areas of expertise and at Cushing's behest, he orchestrated a course in surgical anatomy at the Brigham that enjoyed great popularity among the medical students. These Saturday morning clinics combined anatomic observations with clinical practicalities and became an important part of the curriculum. Cheever made sure his presentations were relevant to the topics underway in their formal courses. For instance, if the students were studying the chest wall, he would present a patient with a breast carcinoma, embellishing the clinical information with a scholarly exposition of breast anatomy and its lymphatic drainage. After a recess, the audience would enter the observation seats above one of the operating rooms, watch the surgery and hear the surgeon elaborate on the structures as they became evident during the procedure.

Crane amusingly describes one "surgical clinic on a topic relating to the [students'] area of dissection. Dr. Cheever was giving such a discussion and demonstration of inguinal hernia. He had a patient with a large indirect inguinal hernia standing in the amphitheatre, trousers and shorts down, while Dr. Cheever, sitting sideways in a straight chair, pointed out the landmarks. In demonstrating the internal inguinal ring he emphasized the importance of having the patient stand and he told the class that some patients underwent a reflex faint when the examiner felt with his index finger deeply into the inguinal canal and that the examiner must be prepared to catch him in his fall. Accordingly, Dr. Cheever felt deeply, the patient fainted and Dr. Cheever caught him."[17]

An unflappable and deliberate surgeon, he performed the most formidable procedures of his day, all anatomically correct and gently executed. He used closed chest massage for cardiac arrest in 1905, a half century before the practice came into routine use. The mortality rate of patients after primary resection of the right colon in the days before antibiotics or adequate transfusions, was comparable to that of the present. His 1936 review of cancer of the colon remained an authoritative statement of the problem for many years. His personal results of surgery for gallstones were the best of his time, while his technique for exploration of the common bile duct has remained standard procedure until the recent advent of endoscopic techniques for the removal of stones.

Although not prolific, his thoughtful, conservative, and precise personality was reflected in his writings, as was his concern for and talent with the English language. His phraseology was exact and his words selected carefully. Several of his articles on medical topics became classics, while essays on more philosophical subjects are models of literary style. For instance, in his presidential address to the American Surgical Association in 1933, *Anatomy Eclipsed*, he waxed pessimistic about the changes occurring in the medical curriculum and the decline in emphasis on the teaching of anatomy. "When a source which for ages has illuminated our steps is eclipsed by another celestial body, it is natural that we should feel disturbed, and even though the newcomer has a radiance of its own, we should inquire whether we are better or worse off, and whether we might not have the benefit of both luminaries to make clear our perilous path. That the anatomy in the medical curriculum has suffered a partial eclipse, and that its obscuration is increasing are so evident that it is incumbent upon those charged with the responsibilities of medical education . . . to examine the situation and register their approval or disapprove of the change which is taking place."[18]

Stately and serious, Cheever was inevitably polite and gentlemanly with an air of Old World gallantry. His relationship with and support of the resident staff was well recognized. His ability to admit his lack of omniscience was reflected in his occasional plaintive pleas for the celestial wisdom of Maurice Richardson when faced with a sick patient with an acute abdomen of uncertain cause. Chilton Crane characterized him further as a "dignified man, of considerable presence, a true patrician, who spoke slowly and carefully. He had gray hair, big ears, and a gray face. He looked a little like a rabbit. Hence the following story. When on visit, (he often alternated with Dr. Homans) he conducted formal afternoon rounds, seeing all the new patients on the surgical service in a revolving bedside visit, with the surgical students and most of the house staff in attendance. The head nurse on the ward would accompany the group, carrying the so called 'rectal tray.'

"The house officer would present the patient by name, complaint and history to Dr. Cheever, who stood at the foot of the bed, fingers intertwined, smiling encouragement to the patient. A patient with a straight forward history of rectal cancer was the subject and the nurse held open the rectal glove for Dr. Cheever and was ready with the lubricant when the patient spoke up with vigor: 'Oh! No! You don't, Old bunnyface. Max Michael (the fourth year student) is my doctor!' "[19]

His loyalty and dedication to surgery gave him membership in many societies and the presidency of several. An enduring sense of responsibility toward Harvard caused him to assume a variety of leadership positions. His interest in scholarship was reflected by his chairmanship of the Boston Medical Library. His careful conservatism and concern with principle promoted his long-term service on the Committee of Ethics of the Massachusetts Medical Society and as an Overseer of the University. But despite an offer of $10,000 to Harvard Medical School if it would accept women, he voted in the minority against the proposal. His stoicism and vigor contributed to his uncomplaining forbearance of progressive arthritis that began in France in World War I and slowly worsened throughout most of his life. During his last few years, the disease made him a virtual prisoner.

WHILE INHALATION ANESTHESIA had gained justifiable stature since its introduction in the middle of the nineteenth century, its use during operative procedures remained perilous for decades thereafter. Based upon his own unfortunate experience as a student at the MGH and because of the relatively high mortality from improper etherization of patients for intra-abdominal procedures during his time at Hopkins, Cushing initiated the use of local anesthesia for several procedures by injecting cocaine into the appropriate nerve roots. Even two decades later John Homans in his *Textbook of Surgery* described the use of "rectal ether anesthesia as a useful substitute for [the more dangerous] anesthesia by inhalation."[20]

One reason for concern was that unsupervised trainees and nurses administered much of the anesthesia in teaching hospitals during the early years of the century. Indeed, the presence of full-time anesthetists on surgical faculties remained a rarity for some decades and evoked intermittent concern. In 1896 at the 50th anniversary celebration of the advent of ether anesthesia, a speaker had commented: "Although the present state of our knowledge leaves much to be desired we may, I think, congratulate ourselves upon the advances which have been made in recent years. With all these additions to our storehouse of knowledge the question may well be asked, 'Why do not deaths from anesthesia show signs of diminution?' The reply is that the responsibilities involved in administering anesthesia are not yet fully realized, that the administration is too often placed in the hands of unskilled men."[21] The new department of surgery at the Brigham faced a similar problem.

Walter Boothby was one of a relatively small group of physicians and dentists beginning to enter positions in anesthesia in the larger institutions.[22] Drawn to the subject as a surgical resident at the Boston City Hospital, he designed an apparatus that would administer a mixture of nitrous oxide and oxygen with or without the addition of ether. He soon formulated the concept of re-breathing to regulate the content of carbon dioxide. In quick succession he refined the technique of intratracheal intubation, described a more effective introducer for a tracheal catheter, initiated the practice of warming anesthetic gases, and originated the idea of a safety valve for the anesthesia machine.

Stimulated by his own interest in the subject, his early involvement with patient monitoring using the ether chart, his insistence on a staff anesthetist to care for his neurosurgical patients, and the desire for an organized program in his new department, Cushing invited Boothby to be supervisor of anesthesia and head of the respiratory research laboratory. In preparation, he arranged that the appointee spend a year in Oxford with the respiratory physiologist J. S. Haldane. The surgeon-in-chief was delighted with this appointment, as he noted in his first *Annual Report* in 1914: "In addition there is a supervisor of anesthesia who personally administers the anesthetics in the most difficult and responsible cases and who happens to be the desirable type of man who gives his full time and has charge of a laboratory for the special study of respiratory problems."[23] Stimulated by the metabolic changes in Cushing's acromegalic patients, Boothby began to examine a series of topics that included basal metabolism, the increasing relationship between pharmacology and anesthesia, mechanical aspects of pulmonary aeration, and the respiratory center of the brain.[24] As the "etherizer" in many of Cushing's intracranial operations, he devised an accurate dosimetry technique for administering and varying the ether-air mixture and measuring ether tension in patients with cerebellar lesions.

In 1916, Boothby accepted a position to organize and run the Metabolism Laboratory at the Mayo Clinic. The war intervened, however, and he joined Cushing in France, ultimately becoming director of the Gas School in Gondrecourt. His later career was filled with observations on basal metabolism and with the development of a mask for oxygen treatment that was soon adapted for pilots at high altitudes. As one of the early specialists in anesthesia, his investigations were far reaching. His departure, however, left a distinct void in the Brigham program.

Cheever, the acting chief during Cushing's absence in France, commented on the loss in the 1916 *Annual Report*. "A valued member of the staff has resigned to accept a post in another institution. This vacancy has not been filled and constitutes one of the pressing needs of the surgical service. A skilled anesthetist to conduct difficult cases and to foster high standards and traditions among the successive groups of house officers is an indispensable factor in successful surgery."[25] He pursued this theme a year later. "A death occurred under ether anesthesia administered for operation for simple hernia. It must be assumed that the death was due to ether, and this has led to a revision of the conditions surrounding the giving of anesthetics. This extremely responsible duty has been entrusted to the most recently appointed group of interns, with the delusion that under the general supervision of the operating surgeon it would be discharged with adequate satisfaction. Time and again the expectation has proved fallacious, although ill-results are usually averted. We have now established the plan of entrusting anesthesia to interns during the second quarter of their terms of service, after they have acquired some clinical judgment and experience; they are instructed by two skilled nurse anesthetists, who themselves conduct the more critical cases."[26]

Despite the early efforts of Cushing and a few of his colleagues in other centers, anesthesia was slow to arrive as an organized specialty in the United States. But the need was increasing as the latitude and complexity of surgery broadened and older and more problematic patients were accepted for operations. The first chair of anesthesia was established at the University of Wisconsin in 1915. While Harvard created its first chair in 1917, it remained vacant until 1936. The rather tenuous position of the specialty during this period may have substantially held back advances such as thoracic and cardiac surgery. This situation was not corrected fully until after World War II.

Cushing brought the urologist, William Quinby, into his new department in 1916. Like the others, he was educated at Harvard then trained in general surgery at the MGH where he allegedly administered the first intravenous infusion at that hospital.[27] Acquiring academic interests early in his residency, he published papers in a variety of subjects including orthopedics, pediatric, and thoracic surgery. Most important for his future career, however, was the period he spent with Hugh Hampton Young, one of Halsted's trainees who had established an innovative and productive urological service at Johns Hopkins. Young was among the first to construct and use the cystoscope, to dilate contracted bladders, to carry out successful perineal prostatectomy, and to remove the obstructing hypertrophied median bar of that gland.

An early figure in his field, Quinby opened a urology service at the Brigham in 1916. Always interested in education, he formed a two-year specialty residency as well as allowing general surgical trainees to rotate through his program. He relied heavily on logic, reasoning, and realism in his approach to his patients, residents and students. "His methods of teaching drew deeply from his own resources and required of his apprentice his best metal. His major contribution as a teacher was an uncanny ability to inspire the student to think—whether he wished to or not?"[28] His studies emphasized concise reasoning and intellectual honesty. Broad interests in applied laboratory science included investigations in vascular and pulmonary surgery in addition to problems of the genitourinary tract. His unabated output of clinical writings in urology included observations on congenital anomalies, cancer, infections, and surgery of the prostate. His treatment of male infertility by re-implantation of the vas deferens brought early attention to this problem.

Quinby published two papers that contributed substantially many years later to the novel subject of renal transplantation at the Brigham. The first, "The function of the kidney when deprived of its nerves," showed that the organ could behave in a completely normal fashion when placed in a different anatomical location in the body.[29] A second,

"The action of diuretics on the denervated kidney" strengthened the initial observation.[30] The information gleaned from these experiments was an important nidus for the events to come.

At the request of the dean and the trustees, he acted as surgeon-in-chief during the period between the death of Cutler and the arrival of Francis Moore. And to his credit, he insisted that physician anesthesiologists care for the patients during surgery, appointing William Derrick as chief of anesthesia to oversee this charge. Training a number of leaders in his field, Quinby was a renowned early figure in urology.

FRANCIS NEWTON WAS CUSHING's final appointment. He joined the staff in 1922 after completing his residency at the Brigham and spending a year abroad visiting surgical clinics in Switzerland. A gentle, conscientious, and soft-spoken individual, he taught generations of residents during the 47 continuous years he remained in the department. Of artistic bent, the beautiful drawings of microscopic anatomy that he began as a medical student were highly sought after by his peers. Never a prolific writer, his legacy was his surgical excellence, often under relatively primitive conditions. "At a time when no specific treatment for sepsis existed, transfusion of 250ml of blood was rare and unpredictable, fluid replacement was by rectal drip and anesthesia had changed relatively little since the time of Morton, the technical performance of the surgical operation very often made the difference between life and death. In this, Francis Newton was an acknowledged master. He was neither fast or slow, but meticulous, precise, gentle and calm. His patients rarely had post-operative sepsis, hemorrhage or shock, and never as a result of his surgical procedure. One surgical generation removed from Halsted, he absorbed his surgical philosophy from Cushing and passed it on to hundreds of students, interns and residents. He never moved so fast that he could not see the flowers."[31]

This group of men accelerated the reputation of the small hospital. By their professional example, efforts and accomplishments they created new generations of surgeons and surgical investigators who, like ever widening ripples in a pond, influenced their own trainees and produced their own disciples.

CHAPTER 5

THE TRANSITION TO
ELLIOTT CUTLER

CUTLER SUCCEEDED Cushing in 1932. With his enthusiasm, efflorescence, and broad surgical interests, he was a different personality type than his more dour and single-minded predecessor. Even at an early age, his peers commented on his ambition and tireless energy, with one friend and admirer later summarizing these lifelong traits in rather poetic hyperbole. "Elliott had always driven the chariot of his busy, feverish life with rein unchecked; not one moment of the day wasted, no evening steeped in *honied* indolence."[1]

Born in Maine, he graduated from Harvard College in 1909, having stroked and captained a victorious varsity crew. First in his class at Harvard Medical School and elected permanent secretary, he spent his final year in pathology with Frank B. Mallory at the Boston City Hospital, then traveled to Germany for an additional period in Ludolph Krehl's surgical pathology laboratory. Taking full advantage of these opportunities and echoing Cushing's own sentiments, he noted their considerable value in his later career. "As I look back on that precious year, it probably did more for me as a budding young medico than any other year in my lifetime, I learned the value of precise work and the importance of making and recording correct observations, and I learned to enter the domain of books, for there is time in the life of the laboratory worker to read and study and thus to become aware of the immense amount of knowledge available to the profession. Moreover, it was this year with Dr. Mallory that led me to spend the next nine months in Krehl's laboratory in Heidelberg, working on a problem that involved pathological disciplines as well as surgery and medicine"[2]

At the end of his internship at the Brigham, he followed Cushing and Boothby to France for three months in 1915 to serve in the Amer-

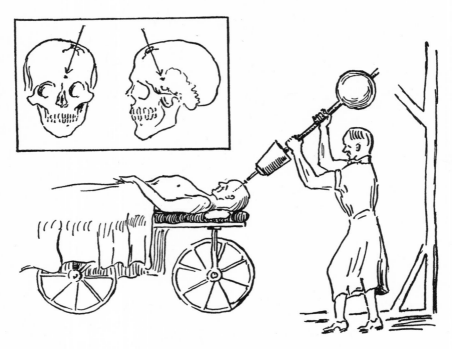

FIGURE 5.1   Cushing's sketch of himself removing a piece of shrapnel from deep in the brain with a magnet. From Cushing H, *From a Surgeon's Journal*, 51.

ican Ambulance Hospital. Cushing later described some of the experiences with his young colleague in Base Hospital Number 5. One example was particularly interesting. With the plethora of head wounds sustained by soldiers imprudently peering over the tops of the trenches in that conflict, the surgeons often had to deal with foreign bodies that had lodged deep in the brain. "The vagaries of the foreign bodies are many. Not only may one find the projectiles themselves, but often pieces of equipment which have been detached and which acquire the full velocity of the bullet itself and are really more dangerous. Sometimes the secondary missiles may have come from someone other than the person it actually hit, even a piece of the skeleton of a neighboring soldier, or a bit of stone or wood."[3] Indeed, a fragment of metallic shell often lay beneath infected bone spicules driven into the cerebral substance. Cushing and Cutler rapidly realized that such missiles should be retrieved and the wounds widely drained, a concept in wound management relatively unaccepted at the time. Concerned that exploration for such fragments by usual surgical means would damage the brain further, the team ingeniously improved an existing magnet to remove them. Cushing described one such instance.

"Several unsuccessful trials this morning to extract the shell fragment by the aid of the magnet from the brain of poor——. I was afraid to use the huge probe which they have. Finally, while I was at lunch, Boothby hit upon precisely what was needed in the shape of a large wire nail about six inches long, the point of which he had carefully rounded off.

"Well, there was the usual crowd in the x-ray room, and approaching corridor, and much excitement when we let the nail slide by gravity into the central mechanism of the smiling patient; for at no time did he have any pressure symptoms, and all of these procedures were without an anesthetic.

"So altogether we finally traipsed into the first floor operating room, where Cutler mightily brings up the magnet, slowly we extract the nail—and—there was nothing on it! More sighs, and people began to go out. A third time—nothing. By this time I began to grumble: 'Never saw anything of this kind pulled off with such a crowd. Hoodooed ourselves from the start. Should have had an x-ray made when the man first entered the hospital.' The usual thing is when one begins to scold his golf balls.

"I had taken off my gloves and put the nail down; but then—let's try just one more! So I slipped the brutal thing again down the tract, three and a half inches to the base of the brain, and again Cutler gingerly swung the big magnet down and made contact. The current was switched on and as before we slowly drew out the nail—and there it was, a little fragment of rough steel hanging on to its tip! Much emotion on all sides."[4]

After an additional year of residency at the MGH upon his return from Europe, Cutler strengthened his academic foundations further by studying with microbiologist Simon Flexner at the Rockefeller Institute in New York City. He recalled the sequence of events. "I [had broken] with tradition when I selected the new Peter Bent Brigham Hospital for my surgical training. This for me was merely the fulfillment of an ambition to work with Dr. Cushing who made, early in my medical school days, an immense personal impression on me. After a year at the Massachusetts General Hospital I again broke with tradition, incurring this time the disapproval of my beloved chief and mentor, Dr. Cushing, by studying immunity under Dr. Simon Flexner. I wished to keep away from the clinic as much as possible so that I could benefit from the stern discipline of a meticulous laboratory worker. I well remember the alarm and even disapproval in the minds of several older surgeons in Boston when I told them I was to study immunity. A leading surgeon of that day asked me for information concerning the topic and told me he had never had cause to use such information in his practice!"[5]

In 1917, again with Cushing, he volunteered for service in France where as chief of professional services in an evacuation hospital, he was awarded the Distinguished Service Medal and a personal citation from General Pershing.[6]

He re-entered the Brigham program in 1919 to spend two years as chief resident, then joined the clinical staff as well as becoming director of the Laboratory for Surgical Research across the street in the medical school quadrangle. He later described his motivations toward an academic career. "It seemed to me that a man in an academic life in the field of surgery must either be interested (1) in technical surgery, (2) in his laboratory investigations, or (3) in the opportunity to educate others in his chosen field. I had long felt that the realm of technical surgery and pure operative surgery could not hold my interest unsupported by other and perhaps more urgent professional ambitions."[7]

Propelled by these professional ambitions and at Cushing's urgings he accepted in 1924 the position of professor of surgery at Western Reserve University School of Medicine in Cleveland and director of the surgical service at Lakeside Hospital. He immediately assumed a pattern of leadership that he retained throughout his career, dedicating many of his energies to the education of young surgeons. They, in turn, remained loyal to him for the remainder of their lives. During his eight years at Lakeside Hospital, Cutler established a training plan for his house staff similar to the one he had learned from his professor and from the traditions of the Brigham.[8]

This strategy was not usual in hospitals throughout the United States during that time, as relatively few programs had embraced Halsted's innovations. It entailed a straight surgical internship in which the residents rotated through given services at 3–4 monthly intervals. Additional assignments included associated fields such as pathology. The resultant five-year pyramidal system rarely posed difficulties at the top, as many of the trainees left to enter private practice, having accrued adequate clinical experience on the way. Cutler also required those remaining as chief residents to spend an extra year or two in the laboratory as added preparation for their university careers. He was careful to instruct these future academicians in the intricacies of scientific writing. "One might note at this time that one of the characteristics that often sets apart a junior member of the staff from his colleagues in a striking fashion is his actual ability to finish and report a piece of work. Teachers who have this matter deeply at heart know how great is the ordeal for the young man to write his first, or even his first dozen, papers. It is common to find eager young men who have good ideas, who are industrious, who will look things up in books, but it is the exceptional man who seems to have that last little push that allows him to get it down on a piece of paper in order to get it into press."[9]

As his philosophy matured, Cutler defined fully his concept of surgical education, emphasizing that all clinical careers, ranging from full-time university-based faculty positions to private practice, could be rewarding, depending on one's motivations. He did, however, differentiate between being a surgeon and becoming a scientist. "One can accept a purely practical or a purely theoretical life and remain a valuable worker in medicine. One may practice the art upon suffering humanity or prosecute the science upon which practice rests, in the absolute solitude of the laboratory. One life is filled with multi-various humanity, with the closest association with men; the other may be as isolated as that of religious hermits who live in mountain caves and reckon their devotion according to their isolation."[10] As Cushing had before him, he decried overspecialization, stressing that an academic surgeon should be trained in the entire existing curriculum and exhorting both senior and junior staff to make surgical teaching as appealing as possible for the students, the best of whom would later apply for an internship. He taught by example, considering "that any arrangement which allows one's pupils to share completely in one's daily work is the most stimulating and satisfactory method of exposition."

He finally discussed the most desirable attributes for a chief of an academic service, emphasizing those he felt his chief residents should develop. "It is certain that this position in surgery requires something more than proficiency in the art. In the physician it requires something beyond the ability to diagnose and treat successfully, and in the surgeon something more than the ability to operate with dexterity and safety. Certainly it requires teaching ability. But, in addition to proficiency in the art and ability to teach, a professor must be one who is also trying to improve the science and art in which he works. We have seen enough of successful practitioners in medicine and surgery who have utilized their teaching positions to increase their practices and who, when they are gone, have left neither pupils, nor work which have furthered the advancement of the field in which they labored." This view has persisted in most teaching programs in academic hospitals throughout the country.

Cutler's long-held dream was to follow his mentor as surgeon-in-chief at the Peter Bent Brigham Hospital. Indeed, in addition to operating on all areas of the body during his tenure in Cleveland he had continued a small neurosurgical practice, perhaps as a measure of expediency. Already elected to the Harvard Board of Overseers in 1927, he explained the lure of returning to Boston in his first *Annual Report*. "The reputations of Harvard University and of the Brigham Hospital were already such as to make it certain I might have more able candidates for a surgical clinic in this hospital than elsewhere. I have the ambition that the Brigham Hospital shall become a more general hospital in the sense that it will treat all forms of disease so that we can emphasize to students, both undergraduate and graduate, the value of a broad general training. In the training of young men, there comes a period when the assumption of great responsibilities becomes one of the most important elements in his continued growth. With such a thought in mind, it is obvious that I should desire that the resident staff should assume a considerable share of the actual work in the operating rooms. This is a Brigham tradition, and my senior colleagues have shown the greatest thoughtfulness in furthering this idea and at the same time in protecting the unusually sick patient by assuming full responsibility in such cases."[11] A committed surgeon, he defended his specialty against the perhaps more obvious forces of those in internal medicine. "Mistakes in surgery may cost the patient his life, whereas a little more rhubarb or jalop hardly does more than hasten the step."[12]

BUT REGARDLESS OF CUTLER'S appointment as his successor, Cushing did not relinquish his position easily. At the beginning of his own tenure at the Brigham two decades before, he and his medical counterpart, Henry Christian, had placed the age of retirement at 63. In fact, when they were setting up the policy, Cushing had written to Christian: "I shall be very glad, for one, to have it legislated to stop active work at sixty. I have an idea that the surgeon's fingers are apt to get a little stiff and thus make him less competent before the physician's cerebral vessels do. However, as I told you, I would like to see the day when somebody would be appointed surgeon somewhere who has no hands, for the operative part is the least part of the work."[13] But despite a rather cursory consideration toward such a step after he turned 60, he did not perform his last surgical operation until two years later, on April 15, 1931, his two-thousandth case of brain tumor.

His appointment as Moseley Professor was to terminate on September 1st, 1932. Eight months before President Lowell of Harvard had written to inform him that Cutler had been chosen over Cheever by a close faculty vote to take over his position. The letter showed a certain level of discomfort. "In accordance with your own preference, Dr. Cutler who was elected your successor by the Corporation was confirmed by the Overseers this afternoon. Now there comes a little awkwardness because we cannot well announce his election so long as you have not formally resigned. You see our embarrassment."[14] Cushing immediately proffered his formal resignation rather huffily,

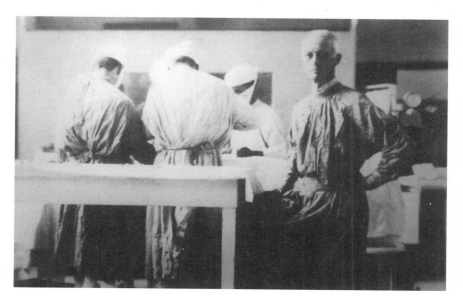

FIGURE 5.2   The 2000th brain tumor operation.

explaining that since his term of service automatically ended toward the end of that year, it had not occurred to him that it was necessary to resign from a position he was not entitled to hold.

Offers of professorships came quickly from several institutions including Lakeside Hospital, Yale, and Hopkins. A rather belated proposal by Edsall and Lowell of a professorship in the history of medicine at Harvard displeased him as too little and too late. In fact Edsall, not overly anxious to keep his irascible colleague in Boston, suggested that Cushing continue to see patients and operate at the nearby Deaconess Hospital as well as to teach the history of medicine at Harvard. The offer did not include a salary, as the proposed incumbent was considered financially well off. No one realized, however, that Cushing had lost considerable capital in the 1929 stock market crash. "His patrimony had been swept away in the financial dither of a banking house whose repute had been thought to have been above reproach. 'I had supposed' he writes to the president of Yale, 'that the trust fund I had established for my family was as secure as anything could legally be, I now learn that the people who had my affairs in hand had so manhandled them that I may have to start afresh as a wage earner.' "[15]

The general recognition by his peers of one of Cushing's greatest contributions assuaged many of the political difficulties and logistical inconveniences of the transition. At age 63, he described a complex polyglandular syndrome caused by basophil adenomas of the pituitary. He had noted over the years that several of his pituitary patients presented with a variety of endocrine abnormalities but never developed the more common visual field defects or increased intracranial pressure. As a result they had not come to surgery. After hearing of two similar instances, he took the opportunity to examine the pituitary of a patient who had suddenly died. Excited by the presence of a basophil adenoma in the gland, he managed to collect a few other cases. All showed the same lesions. His definitive paper on the subject in 1932 received wide acclaim.[16] Members of the newly formed Harvey Cushing Society quickly christened the condition Cushing's Disease.

Although most of his friends and supporters were delighted with the change in his life, an underlying sense of loss occasionally surfaced. "What a wonderful opportunity Cutler will have as compared with the situation that you faced some years ago. He is no doubt the most promising man of his age in surgical America. I cannot view your retirement at Harvard with complacency. Your influence on world medicine and particularly your stimulation of scientific ideals and accomplishments must continue with increasing power for many many years. It would be wonderful if you could see your way clear to go to Baltimore and there create a veritable Mecca for historically-minded pilgrims. Somehow or other I cannot see you retiring from surgery and any plan that you contemplate should incorporate in it two or three days each week which you will devote to your chosen surgical field. Heaps of us depend upon you for that rare encouragement which only you can give."[17]

Returning to the Brigham after spending the summer in Europe, Cushing found that Cutler had moved into his office in his absence, having first emptied it of all its contents. The new chief had also rearranged the operating schedule and taken over management of the surgical clinic. Assigned a room elsewhere and relieved of all responsibilities, Cushing continued his studies on meningiomas with Louise Eisenhardt, a long-term collaborator in charge of his pathologic specimens. Relatively forgotten by those in the hospital, he embraced the chance to accept the Sterling Professorship of Neurology at Yale arranged through John Fulton, his fellow bibliophile, long-term disciple, and principal biographer. But as one of the surgical house staff noted a few years later: "We [Harvard medical students] were not particularly interested in neurosurgery. In fact, we really had no great interest in Cushing, although we knew he was famous and had contributed a great deal [to the school]."[18] On October 12, 1933, "he escaped [from the Brigham] through a side door."[19] Eisenhardt went with him.

With the Sterling Chair and a handsome salary, Cushing thrived in New Haven. He had brought all of his books and papers. The vast collection of brain tumors that he had collected over decades became the core of the Brain Tumor Registry. Surrounded by the records of his life's work and with congenial companions, he lived happily and productively until his death in 1939. He never returned to Boston.

Cushing's negative feelings about what he considered his poor treatment by the Brigham and by Harvard Medical School lasted through at least one more generation of his family. Many years later, I had become director of the Surgical Research Laboratory. During the 1980s I was trying to raise money for the ongoing investigations there. I sent several articles that I had published about Cushing to one of his daughters with a lengthy discourse about her father's interest in and

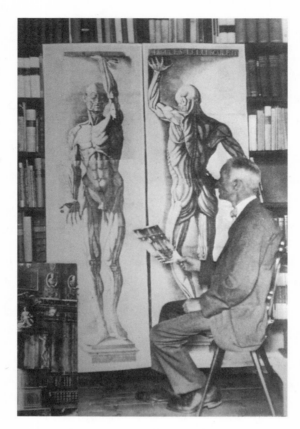

FIGURE 5.3   Cushing examining Cattani's anatomical engravings, Bologna, 1929.
From Thomson EH, *Harvey Cushing: Surgeon, Author, Artist*, 271.

support of the Harvard laboratory, explaining our current need for funds. A polite note came to me shortly thereafter, explaining that she "couldn't see her way clear for a donation at this time." Two days later we read in the newspaper that she had endowed two Cushing Chairs at Yale. Harvard was left empty handed. One sporting observer suggested that Yale had fallen on the ball that Harvard fumbled.

As honors continued to flood in from all over the world, Cushing spent many of his energies in planning his library at Yale.[20] This idea started gradually. Following a visit to the Osler Library at McGill, he wrote enthusiastically to his friend and book collector, Arnold Klebs, about his plan. 'As I may have intimated to you in times past I have always intended to have a checklist of my books made and then to have them sold so that others might have the pleasure of collecting them as I have done. This idea began to wane in favor of leaving them to Yale to be kept together as the basis of a medicohistorical collection. I have talked the matter over with John [Fulton]. I gather that he would like to leave his books also when the time comes, making a Fulton-Cushing collection. I woke up in the middle of the night with the thought—why not a Klebs-Fulton-Cushing collection so that we three could go down in bibliophilic posterity hand in hand."[21] After prolonged organizational and financial difficulties, the university finally approved of a new building to house the collection. Cushing was delighted to learn about this a few hours before his death in 1939. Fulton's books joined the collection in 1940 and Klebs's arrived from Denmark after the end of World War II.

Cutler graciously acknowledged the contribution of his predecessor in the 1932 *Annual Report*, written in his first year as Surgeon-in-Chief. "I am taking the opportunity of incorporating in these reports a notice of the deep appreciation which all who have ever served this institution must have for my predecessor. It is impossible for me to write down my personal feelings toward Dr. Cushing. His pupils know of our relationship, of my deep devotion to his great abilities which he has so liberally given to his pupils in these 20 years. No one in this country has achieved a similar position, unless it may be said that Dr. Halsted left his mantle for his pupil, Harvey Cushing. The characteristics of these two men were quite different, their abilities and ambitions obviously widely separated, and yet they both proved themselves to be of the quality from which great teachers are made. That the people who have held such high positions should be dissimilar leaves hope to others who have similar ambitions. Indeed, it may be important that successful individuals have quite distinct characteristics in order to achieve success for their institutions."[22]

CUTLER'S DYNAMISM AND ENERGY infected all around him. His sense of the dramatic was finely honed. Tall and athletic, he invariably ran up stairs and raced down the corridors of the hospital, occasionally vaulting over a hospital laundry cart if it seemed in his way. He always seemed short of time, moving quickly "with the tails of his long white coat often wind borne."[23] His specially fitted blue surgical scrubs worn under a white coat suggested a press of events, as if he was needed in

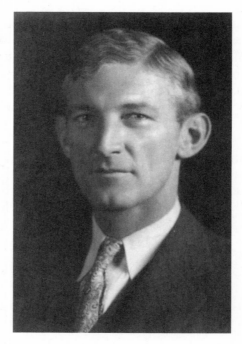

FIGURE 5.4   Elliott Cutler.

the operating room, and allowed him the opportunity to change to his usual dark suits in his office as necessary. He even transmitted this aura of urgency to the students at his eight o'clock lectures; his often slightly delayed arrival at the podium gave extra significance to his presence.

A student later described the teaching atmosphere that he and his staff engendered. He "had assembled a group of talented and for the most part likeable doctors. These young surgeons clearly were inspired by, and emulated [the professor]. They liked us students and gave generously of their time, an experience I had not had at the MGH or Boston City Hospital. Rounds were interesting and challenging. Cutler liked to teach informally, and his use of hyperbole to get across a point was unforgettable. Once, when one of my classmates was holding a retractor in the skull of one of the patients, he must have become tired after standing long in an uncomfortable position, and Cutler said: 'Don't pull on that brain, boy, it's just water.' Within days this remark was known to every student at the school, and it made an indelible impression."[24]

Cutler's lengthy and diverse bibliography mirrored his protean surgical interests. Several early surgical concepts were his, arising from unsolved clinical problems and embellished and expanded by laboratory experiments. He was the first in the United States to describe the threat of pulmonary embolism as a postoperative complication, hypothesizing that such emboli formed at the operative site itself but not appreciating that many venous thromboses originate in the legs. The possibilities of operative relief of a variety of cardiac abnormalities intrigued him for years and challenged his surgical expertise.

He believed implicitly that a sound basis of surgical technique should be taught by example to those in training, based particularly on his adherence to Halsted's methods of careful hemostasis and gentleness in dissecting tissues. A master surgeon, "smooth, gentle, graceful, no hesitation, no false move, he handled instruments with the delicacy

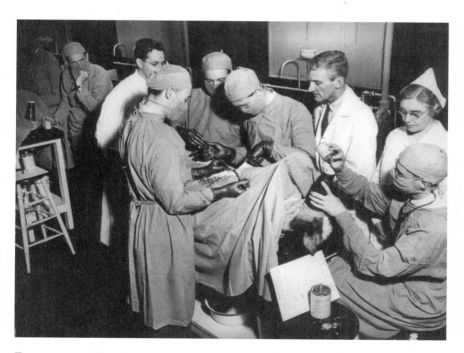

Figure 5.5   The Course in Aseptic technique in full swing in 1938. Cutler and Walter are instructing the students. Francis Moore, anesthetist, casts a jealous eye on the proceedings from the next table.

93

of a portrait painter with his brush."[25] Equally at home performing complex neurosurgical procedures as he was in the thorax or abdomen, he was the acknowledged leader of the surgical team, fully in charge, never distraught, teaching exuberantly, and making his operations enjoyable experiences for his students and residents. His operative field was often a lesson in anatomy. "His ambition to improve the practice of surgery, to extend his confines and to inspire his students to pursue its science and art was the object of his incredible energy." His responsibility toward his patients extended far beyond the peri-operative period.

Cutler's dedication to teaching and to his students did not limit itself to addresses and publications but was manifest both in clinical conferences and in weekly laboratory meetings where, over tea and biscuits, he and his research fellows would listen and criticize presentations of ongoing work.[26] Spending much time with the students in the laboratory course in aseptic technique, he stressed independent thinking, scientifically controlled research, and clear communication of experimental results to colleagues. An eloquent apologist for vivisection, he believed that the surgical laboratory was the place where clinical problems could be defined and solved in relevant animal models.[27] His own productivity and conversance with many facets of his discipline inspired many of his trainees to enter careers in academic surgery. They not infrequently assumed chairmanships of departments in major universities.

One of Cutler's principal contributions was the *Atlas of Surgical Operations* co-authored with his Brigham colleague, Robert Zollinger.[28] Its aim was uniform: the benefit of the surgical patient through well considered, effective, and standardized operative techniques. This large book showed each surgical procedure in a step-by-step fashion via clear and accurate pen-and-ink drawings. On the opposite page was a concise description of each figure, with a brief discussion of indications and pre-operative preparation. Mildred Codding, an artist who had trained at Hopkins under Max Brödel and had worked with Cushing for years, produced the drawings over a three-year period. Standing behind Cutler in the operating room through many of his operations, she carefully sketched the salient aspects of the procedures. This book went through six editions and taught generations of surgeons. "It was his 'Atlas' which was devoted to bringing greater safety to the surgical patient by having operations done more accurately and effectively."[29]

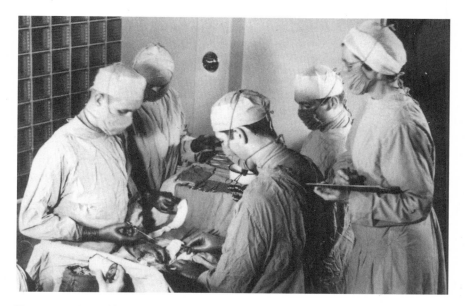

Figure 5.6   Mildred Codding, the surgical artist, at work.

Regardless of the traditions, accomplishments, and worldwide reputation that the Brigham had gained under his predecessor, Cutler quickly discovered that he had inherited a rundown physical plant with unaddressed problems ranging from infrastructural defects to inadequate finances. "There was an administration who persistently worshiped the architectural perfection of a 20-year-old hospital designed at turn of the century concepts and [with the] technology of a sanitarium. Impoverished by the Great Depression and overburdened by indigent patients, the hospital was struggling to survive."[30] Indeed, there were discussions about closure.

And at least one visiting European surgeon was less than sanguine in his impression of its efficiency and organization. "The Peter Bent Brigham is disorderly and in part unhygienic, because there is not the same washing and scrubbing as we are used to in our hospitals. There are employed nurses without number, with their helpers and helpers' helpers in the form of lady typists and stenographers, secretaries, keepers of the lists, and more. One must not suppose this to be some manifestation of the so-called speed and efficiency of America. On the contrary, these storied faculties, said to be part and parcel of America, was something of which I saw little or nothing at the Peter Bent Brigham Hospital. Never have I seen a hospital where there was such a dalliance with time and so much flirtation between nurses and doctors. Operations posted and scheduled to begin at 9:00 a.m. were not underway before 10:30 a.m. The pace was leisurely in the extreme— not merely in the brain operations, which always must proceed with circumspection and deliberation, but also in general surgery such as appendectomies."[31]

Even the ebullient Cutler became discouraged, describing some of the problems he and his department had to endure in his 1938 *Annual Report*. "We have almost no provision for adequate bacteriology, which is the very basis for surgical practice. When one considers the surgical building, we face the same issues. The quarters have been unchanged since 1913, the original type of sterilizers are still in use . . . Sterile instruments must be carried across a corridor used by visitors and patients. Advances in anesthetic apparatus find us unequipped since we cannot afford such expensive items. The quarters originally assigned for the recovery of patients have to be utilized for storage of apparatus. We have spread into the wings of the amphitheater for the care of the recovery period of our patients. We use poorly sharpened knives since we cannot afford the best type available. If we wish to buy a simple piece of apparatus, such as an underwater electrical scalpel, it takes months of careful consideration to find the small amount [of money] to pay for it. We have to set up in our operating rooms sterile supplies for the whole plant and thus crowd our operating room nurses for the great labor when their minds and time should be concerned with the care of the patient whose life is jeopardized at the operating table. Somehow we must find space for a central surgical supply and sterilizing plant. The making up of surgical supplies and sterilization is not a task for the operating room personnel. In the same space should also be centered the manufacture and sterilization of fluids for intravenous and subcutaneous use now carried out in space generously donated by [the] pathology [department], but by this very necessity, further crippling this splendid department."[32] The years leading into World War II were indeed difficult.

One of the more dramatic manifestations of the infrastructural defects that Cutler faced almost upon his arrival at the Brigham was that many of the patients and staff alike were affected intermittently by bouts of diarrhea. He christened this affliction, "the squitters." Ironically, Carl Walter, a new intern supported strongly by his chief resident Robert Zollinger and then by Cutler himself, solved this engineering aberation as he was to solve many others during the course of his career. His first clue to the trouble was that the drinking water turned blue. He tells the story.

"The furor began on a Sunday evening when I infused gallbladder dye intravenously for a Graham Test. The patient's room was on the top floor of the private pavilion. He promptly suffered a severe pyrogen reaction. I immediately stopped the infusion. The solution had been prepared in the hospital pharmacy. The burette, rubber tubing and needle had been sterilized in the bedpan sterilizer in the ward utility room. I discarded the deep purple dye remaining in the burette into the bedpan hopper along with the contents of a second bottle of dye intended for another patient then gravitated to the Doctors Dining Room on the first floor of an adjoining building for a bedtime snack. I was amazed to see purple water in the steam table in the serving counter and spilling from the drinking fountain in the dining room.

"The following dawn on rounds with Elliott Cutler I dumped methylene blue into the same bedpan hopper and led him to the drinking fountain to demonstrate the likely cause of the squitters—an obvious shunt between the sewer system and the water supply. Complexities arose at lunch time when it was discovered that the vanilla ice cream made in the kitchen below the dining room was blue. When the ice man began to refill the ice boxes on the various nursing units he noticed that the 350 pound blocks of ice that had been frozen overnight in the ice making department next to the kitchen were blue.

"That an intern had demonstrated the cause of the squitters was irrelevant to the emergency session of the Executive Committee [which] convened to mete out discipline for bringing ridicule to the hospital. However, the need for sanitary plumbing demonstrated that day resulted in the replacement of the cold water piping system throughout the sprawling hospital. Even after a new water system of copper pipe was installed, including vacuum breakers at each fixture, the Yankee superintendent did not forgive either the upstart intern or his mentor—Zollinger. This despite the fact that he, himself, no longer had to lug pails of water from the main floor of his home on the hospital grounds to flush the toilets in the second floor bathrooms."[33]

WITH THE ENTRANCE of the United States into World War II, Cutler again joined the Army between 1942 and 1945 to serve as the chief surgical consultant in Europe. With his new rank of brigadier general, he brought many of his residents and junior faculty with him to General Hospital No. 5. This was eventually divided into two hospitals, one for the European Theater, the other for the Pacific. His men served in both. He and Zollinger devised the portable surgical hospital (the precursor of the MASH unit introduced by Michael DeBakey during the Korean War), in time for the Normandy invasion. He orchestrated the orderly removal and care of casualties, an important contribution.

His ambassadorial talents became finely honed as he visited every medical outpost in Europe, directing and inspiring those working there. On a surgical mission to Russia toward the end of the war, Cutler's obvious admiration of their surgical achievements and friendliness strengthened a cordial, albeit short-lived, relationship between the two countries who were then allies.[34] His wide acquaintanceship with colleagues in many countries increased his renown. "The slight, erect, soldierly figure, the unvarying bon amie, attractive voice and charming smile made Elliot Cutler a veritable Paladin, and one of the most wonderful ambassadors of surgery the world has known."[35] For his services, he received a second Distinguished Service Medal, The Order of the British Empire, the Croix de Guerre, and the Order of Haakon VII from Norway. His two Distinguished Service Medals from two World Wars are honors still unique among medical officers.

CHAPTER 6

"PA CUTLER'S BOYS"

T HE GENERAL SURGICAL faculty was well established when Cutler arrived at the Brigham, with Homans, Cheever, Quinby, and Newton executing the bulk of the operative procedures and carrying out most of the teaching of the house staff. Each of them continued to fulfill their various departmental duties effectively during the period that the professor and most of his juniors were absent during World War II. Despite the substantial disruption of the conflict, the reputation of the professors and the senior staff left behind plus the influence of those at the Children's Hospital across Shattuck Street continued to encourage highly competent applicants to enter the surgical program.

The improvements in patient care that emerged primarily from treatment of the wounded changed medicine and its associated sciences dramatically in the post-war period, often in ways not visualized by the older practitioners. A new range of pharmaceutical agents, most notably penicillin, was becoming available. With advances in anesthesia, increasing capabilities for blood transfusion, operative innovations and peri-operative monitoring, surgeons were honing their skills in the repair or reconstruction of diseased or injured body areas that they hitherto had not considered.

At the same time, public expectations and desires for medical and scientific knowledge were increasing. Cutler enumerated the new currents beginning to swirl around his profession. "1) the great extension of life in recent years, due largely to man's knowledge of the role of bacteria in infectious diseases and hence how to avoid infections; (2) the recent successful attacks on other types of diseases, as seen in the present methods of treatment for diabetes and pernicious anemia; (3) the rapid progress of surgical therapy to the point where a majority of our citizens have at some time benefited from this form of treatment; and (4) the recent experiments emphasizing the tremendous roles that minute quantities of chemical substances, known as hormones or vitamins, may play in life—all give evidence that modern medicine is indeed one of the most brilliant movements in applied science."[1] Reacting to these new forces, he soon found that he had to enlarge his faculty and broaden his department beyond its existing scope.

Franc Ingraham was already in place during the transition between chiefs. Cushing had ensured a smooth continuum in neurosurgery as he neared retirement by appointing him to the staff in 1929. Ingraham had trained with Cushing at the Brigham with the exception of a research period spent with neurosurgeon Walter Dandy at Johns Hopkins and a year at Oxford in the physiology laboratories of Sir Charles Sherrington.[2] While in England, he collaborated with John Fulton, a younger colleague who was to become his brother-in-law.

An exquisite and careful technician, Ingraham directed his energies increasingly toward the novel field of neurological surgery in children.[3] As the study of potentially reparable problems unique to the developing nervous system was relatively unexplored, he expended much effort in conceptualizing, defining, and correcting such abnormalities. Emboldened by the excellence of his results and those of his trainees, neurosurgeons around the United States increasingly accepted his innovations in the operative treatment of such diverse conditions as subdural hematoma in infants, subdural effusions secondary to bacterial meningitis in infancy, congenital spina bifida and its various manifestations, premature closure of the cranial sutures, classification and treatment of hydrocephalus, and the special problems relating to prolonged intracranial procedures in children.[4] He investigated the influence of body growth as a modifying factor in surgery of the central nervous system and emphasized the importance of improving and arresting progressive neurological deficits in relatively asymptomatic children to control their late effects.

Ingraham cared for neurosurgical patients both at the Brigham and at the adjacent Children's Hospital during Cutler's absence during the war, encouraging a combined specialty-training relationship between the two hospitals. Refurbishing a previously underutilized laboratory, he and his group first used the newly available adrenocorticotrophic hormone (ACTH), elaborated by the pituitary gland and acting on the adrenal cortex, and the adrenal hormone, cortisone, as adjuncts to operations on pituitary and parapituitary tumors. This experience presaged the universal application of cortico-steroids in controlling brain swelling. Later, in response to combat needs, he collaborated with colleagues at the medical school in developing hemostatic fibrin foam and fibrin film, a concept perhaps based on the muscle pledgets that Cushing had introduced years before for bleeding of the brain. As by-products of the blood fractionation program ongoing at the medical school and sponsored by the U.S. Navy, these substances proved valuable in treating war wounds and in various types of civilian surgery. They were the precursors of gelatin foam, a hemostatic material now used routinely.

A productive member of many societies and editorial boards, his peers held Ingraham in high esteem. Although quiet in manner, he was a superb teacher with a penchant for attracting and stimulating young men of ability and energy to work with him. His contributions to pediatric neurosurgery initiated an important subspecialty that was

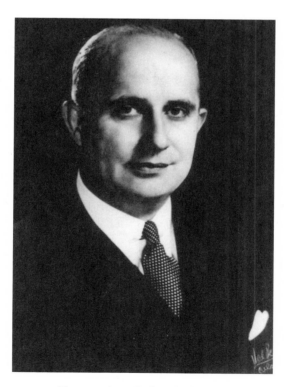

Figure 6.1   Robert Zollinger.

to be carried forward in the next generation of Brigham surgeons by his successor, Donald Matson. From their unique and innovative experience at the neurosurgical unit at Children's Hospital came the 1954 publication of their classic monograph, *Neurosurgery in Infancy and Childhood.*[5]

OTHER MEMBERS OF THE FACULTY were less established. A number of young surgeons, "Pa Cutler's boys," had joined the staff for relatively short periods before leaving for wartime service. Cutler had brought several of these individuals with him from Lakeside to complement and enrich those already in the Brigham program. Robert Zollinger was one of the most visible. He first met Cutler in Cleveland in 1927 as a senior medical student at Ohio State University, having already been accepted as a surgical intern by Cushing. Following his residency at Lakeside, he moved back with his professor to the Brigham as chief resident. Despite his forthright and direct personality, the Mid-westerner had to endure some teasing by his East Coast colleagues. "The Harvard residents asked me, 'What did they teach you at Ohio State, Zollinger, culture or agriculture? I told them "Quiz me, you SOBs, and find out!' "[6]

Despite these imprecations, he remained there for nine years except for a period as commanding officer of the 5th General Hospital in Europe. His influence immediately became apparent. A stern leader, he instilled discipline, precision, and dedication into his junior colleagues, while at the same time enlivening the team with his well-honed sense of humor. Chilton Crane, one of his fellow residents, gives an example of Zollinger's teaching technique. "His no nonsense approach to patient work-ups and his efficiency in promoting good patient care despite the hazards imposed by the teaching phases of a residency training program [can be seen in the following episode]. A resident on the private wards was given responsibility for operating on the public ward patients with acute appendicitis. This resident (T. B. Quigley, in fact) was starting the usual McBurney incision with Zolly watching from a small viewing stand in OR No.1. The procedure was going very slowly with much hesitation. 'Get moving! Pick up the knife and cut!' was the order from the stands. This was shortly followed by an overly energetic cut into the caecum. Dr. Zollinger then gave all the appropriate instructions for caecal repair before the appendix was removed and he followed the benign postoperative course with care."[7]

Carl Walter elaborated further. "Devotion to patients, perfecting surgical skills, increasing clinical acumen, curiosity for clinical investigation and a compelling love for teaching characterized Robert Zollinger. I came to respect, admire and emulate two attributes. First, as a teacher, Zolly goaded students to learn to be a doctor. He was an instructor-educator-trainer with a humorous flair for coaching that often bordered on the outrageous. His unforgettable impact yanked mediocrity out of surgical behavior and instilled a determination to excel. Each trainee discovered his potential as a clinician at a period when surgical intervention was supported by elementary physiology and meager diagnostic technology. Stoups, compresses, poultices, hot soaks, clysters, bed rest and fresh air dominated bedside surgical therapy. Second, he possessed the mark of the true academician. He tolerated deviation of individual students from a rigid training program, and extended encouragement and support for such tangential effort. When these violate institutional narcissism, the most dedicated chief resident may harbor doubts. Zolly's tolerance was a prime example of scholarship at its best."[8]

Zollinger's care of his patients, love of teaching, operative prowess, and enthusiasm for clinical investigation were highly regarded. He carried out several early studies on gastric and biliary surgery in dogs; his technique (with Charles Branch) of dilating the papilla of Vater influenced substantially surgery of the common bile duct in patients. In 1947 he became chairman of surgery at Ohio State. Continuing in that position for three decades, he remained a highly visible leader of American surgery throughout his career.

J. Englebert Dunphy was another important member of the general surgical staff during Cutler's tenure, having trained at the Brigham and worked in the Surgical Research Lab as a Cabot Fellow. After Army service he combined clinical practice with research interests, soon reporting the first successful autotransplantation of the adrenal gland in dogs. With K. N. Udupa, later to become Chancellor of Vaneras Hindu University in India, his early studies on the physiology of wound healing presaged eventual investigations into collagen chemistry of that phenomenon.[9] His observations on the pathology of experimental traumatic shock and its correction by the infusion of bovine serum albumin complemented a significant effort by chemists at the medical school.

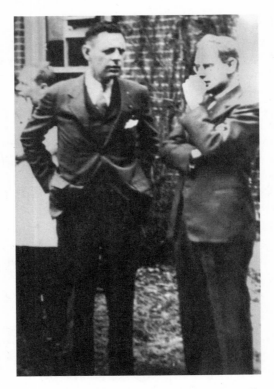

FIGURE 6.2   Thomas Quigley and Bert Dunphy.

One of these, Edwin J. Cohn, had established a Laboratory of Physical Chemistry at Harvard Medical School in 1920 to characterize protein structure, a departure from established traditions of the time.[10] In December 1941 the government appropriated his entire supply of pure human albumin to treat those injured during the attack of Pearl Harbor. As the war progressed, the demands of the wounded caused Cohn's laboratory to expand into a factory. Plasma was fractionated from vast quantities of blood using Carl Walter's new separation apparatus and obtained largely through Walter's efforts with the Red Cross. Plasma fractions, both bovine and human, were tested on prisoners and on medical students. Carried out before the days of human subject committees, these experiments were not without flaw. Two prisoners died of serum sickness from the animal protein. The students were admitted to the Brigham, bled into shock then resuscitated with the human material, in part based on Dunphy's findings in dogs. Newly available gamma globulin, another serum fraction, was used to prevent measles and eventually to attenuate the effects of polio. The collaboration between chemists and clinicians and between physicians and surgeons contributed substantially to the war needs.

Crane recalls an example of Dunphy's rather original personality. "A remarkable man who gained several high positions through his own home grown abilities, and hard work, strengthened by his Jesuit faith— and greatly promoted by an exuberant personality and a rollicking, occasionally hardball sense of humor. An example of this last went as follows. The senior resident on the ward service was responsible for seeing surgical consultations at the Boston Psychopathic Hospital, almost next door. Dunphy was the chief surgical resident and the senior resident involved who shall be nameless was brusque and arrogant and generally disliked. A call came to Dr. Cutler's office from the Psychopathic Hospital about a patient there with subacute abdominal pain. Would the surgeon see him? Of course. Dunphy was given the message which he passed on to his junior. Just before he left, Dunphy called the Psychopathic in some distress. He said that a schizophrenic postoperative hernia patient, on C-Main, who liked to pose as a doctor, had overheard the conversation about the consultation at their hospital. He had taken a resident's white coat from the clean laundry basket and slipped out the side door onto the tennis courts according to a nurse who thought he was a resident. If Dunphy's guess was correct and he showed up at the Psychopathic, they should have some strong guards grab him and put him in confinement because he could be quite dangerous. Accordingly, he [the resident] was jumped and thrown into a padded cell. About 10 minutes later, Dunphy called the Psychopathic back to report that the schizophrenic hernia patient had returned to the ward voluntarily and that they should not worry about him. 'Locked up? My God what a terrible mistake! Let him go and see the patient.' "[11] One can only guess the explanations given.

He invariably leavened his sense of duty with wit. Donald Matson recalled when he and a fellow intern approached Dunphy, the chief resident, for an evening off. Having worked very hard and not being off duty for a long time, they requested permission to go to the theater in Boston to see a new show. He gazed at the pair for a long moment, shook his head and noted: "Well, if you really want to miss all that's going on here in the hospital for a whole evening, you can go." In another instance, Matson queried his senior about the one-week vacation allotted to the house staff each year. Again he looked dubious and suggested: "Well, Don, go if you want to. But after all, you are only going to be here for seven years."[12]

Dunphy remained at the Brigham for several years before assuming the first of several chairmanships and major leadership positions in surgery in the United States. His later papers on hospice care and death and dying have become classics. I vividly remember my own later experience with him. Seeking a surgical internship during my final year of medical school, I traveled around the country for interviews. He was chairman at the University of Oregon at the time. Following a substantial and nervous-making delay, I was ushered into his presence. Among other subjects we discussed was my Harvard background. The conversation finished with his comment: "Young man, the only difference between Harvard and the University of Oregon is that at Harvard there are many people like me, and here there is only one." I still have not thought of an appropriate riposte!

HARTWELL HARRISON, ANOTHER MEMBER of Cutler's staff, was a joyous, charming, and charismatic son of Virginia, its university and its medical school. Following his internship under Cutler at Lakeside Hospital in 1932 he came to the Brigham for the remainder of his surgical and urological training. He served in Australia and New Guinea during the war, correlating dehydration with the high incidence of renal stones among the troops and, in the years before antibiotics, initiating a program of fever therapy for soldiers who had contracted gonorrhea. He published widely on the hormonal changes in the aging male, prostate cancer and the effect of endocrine ablation on its rate of progression, diseases of the adrenal gland, renal ischemia, and renal hypertension. A master of surgical technique and a highly-visible member of the original transplant team, he removed the kidney from the first identical twin donor in 1954, then assumed responsibility for all living donors in the years to come. He was a gregarious and popular figure, taking much personal interest in his trainees and operating room staff, and developing and sustaining an enduring urology resident education program among several hospitals in the region. He remained at the Brigham for half a century, serving as chief of urology for three decades.

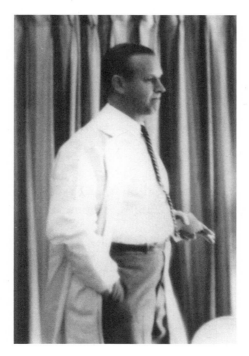

FIGURE 6.3   Hartwell Harrison.

Cushing's interest in the pituitary and pituitary-adrenal axis endured at the Brigham for many years and in many guises. Harrison pursued the subject with one of his more important contributions, surgery of the adrenal gland. The study stemmed from his close collaboration with George Thorn, newly appointed as chief of medicine. Thorn was investigating the physiologic effects of the adrenal cortical hormones, an emerging subject that was generating much potential interest in the treatment of several disease states. Investigations into these substances had accelerated during the war in response to an erroneous rumor that the Germans had developed an adrenal hormone that could increase the performance of soldiers beyond their normal limitations of fatigue and stress. Scientists at the Mayo Clinic, then at the Upjohn and Merck companies, identified and produced a series of steroids. One of these, progesterone, was found to be abundant in a Mexican yam; cortisol could be easily synthesized from it. Other hormones of various structures and of various functions followed which provided tools to examine unique facets of human physiology.

By 1950 Thorn and a junior associate, John Merrill, had made several observations which were soon to involve Harrison, Joseph Murray, and other members of the surgical staff. One of these was that administration of deoxycorticosterone, a salt retaining adrenal hormone, could aggravate hypertensive cardiovascular disease.[13] The investigators had also noted that the elevated blood pressure of hypertensive patients would decline to subnormal levels if they subsequently developed adrenal insufficiency, Addison's Disease. Cardiovascular abnormalities associated with the condition, particularly enlargement of the heart, reversed themselves.[14] Administration of maintenance doses of deoxycorticosterone caused the blood pressure of these affected individuals to increase to abnormally high levels while cortisone, a non-salt retaining steroid, not only reduced blood pressure to normal but reversed other abnormalities. With this background, Harrison performed the first bilateral total adrenalectomy in severely hypertensive patients, approaching the glands through the back.[15] Treated with appropriate steroid combinations their hypertension normalized and they did well. Not only was this a clinical triumph, it set the stage for the use of steroids in transplant patients.

Long on the board of trustees and an enthusiastic and loyal alumnus of the University of Virginia, one of Harrison's deep desires was to be buried on its campus. Upon his death, Mrs. Harrison contacted the Chancellor of the University for permission, only to be summarily informed that the only person ever buried on its hallowed grounds was Thomas Jefferson himself.[16] Not one to be so easily defeated by university officialdom, she put together a bag that contained her husband's ashes, a sandwich, and a trowel, and flew to Virginia. Sitting on the lawn, she ate her lunch, dug a hole beneath a tree and buried the ashes.

Before World War II, many general surgeons specialized in the care of fractures. Carl Walter was one of them. Thomas Quigley was another. Educated at Harvard, he trained at the Brigham under Cutler before becoming chief of orthopedics in the 5th General Hospital in Europe. One of his colleagues in the department of surgery, Richard Warren, amusingly described his first encounter with his colleague during the war as he (Warren) stepped onto English soil from the troop ship that had carried him from New York. Captain Quigley, always dramatic, had been in Britain for several months and was play-ing the role of the "English officer" to the hilt, wearing tall, shiny boots, a tightly belted uniform, a white scarf, and carrying a swagger stick. Warren was incredulous.

Returning as surgeon for the Harvard Department of Athletics, he was for years a well-recognized fixture at football games, wearing a red beret, pacing the sidelines, and running onto the field to examine the injured. Interested particularly in trauma and athletic injuries, he mapped out a comprehensive means of treating the special needs of the athlete and organized a national approach to sports injuries. A colorful figure on the wards, he stimulated many residents to enter orthopedics. Proud of his general surgical training, however, he refused to join the specialty despite repeated offers of the privilege by the orthopedic establishment. Indeed, he became editor of the broadly based *American Journal of Surgery*. His interest in acting and well-developed sense of melodrama had given him the opportunity, years before, to appear on stage with Henry Fonda and James Stewart. These thesbian propensi-ties showed in his professional life. "His pungent wit, precision, and intrinsic dramatic ability made him a colorful, effective lecturer, and bedside teacher."[17]

In his later years, perforation of a sigmoid diverticulum necessi-tated a partial resection of his large bowel, and creation of a temporary colostomy. Predictably, he suffered a variety of complications despite heroic care by Francis Moore and his staff. During his recuperation, Quigley penned an unforgettable poem to his surgeons, entitling it:

Lines in praise of the sphincter muscle written while enduring a tempo-rary colostomy and Respectfully dedicated to Doctors Thomas Botsford and Francis Moore.

"Of all the muscles in the carcass
The one least praised lies hid in darkness,
Sensing gas and fluid pressure
In times of stress and also leisure.
At moments private and sedate
Wondrous music it can make,
From deepest bass to C sharp minor
(Few trombones are any finer).
But when social custom doth decree

Silent zephyrs it can free.
Recognition then is poor;
Rarely can one spot the doer.
O noble myofibril ring
At last I saw thy praises sing.
This present anarchistic vent
Sheltered in its plastic tent
Hath no pucker for control.
It's just an ordinary Hole."

Surgery of the blood vessels has been a consistent departmental interest throughout its history, enriched by Homans's work on venous and lymphatic obstruction, Robert Gross's correction of congenital

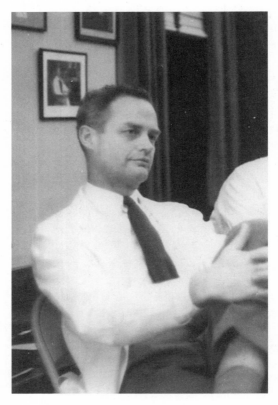

FIGURE 6.4   Richard Warren.

vascular anomalies in children and novel means, with Charles Huf-nagel, to preserve adult arteries for later use, Warren's and Crane's investigations into both arterial and venous disease, and John Man-nick's innovative reconstructions and repair of abnormal vessels.

Despite the limitations that existed both in the techniques and con-cepts of vascular repair and reconstruction after World War II, Richard Warren and Chilton Crane returned to the Brigham from the conflict ready to pursue this topic. Warren was from a long line of Boston surgeons: one ancestor served in the Revolutionary War; another, John Collins Warren, performed the first successful operation under anesthesia at the MGH in 1846; a third, J. Collins Warren, was the first Moseley Professor of Surgery at Harvard and was heavily involved in the gestation and birth of the Brigham Hospital. After graduating from Harvard College, Richard Warren studied classics at Trinity College, Cambridge, an experience that gave him the facility and motivation to translate Latin poetry for pleasure during much of his life. Training in surgery at the MGH, the Brigham, and the University of Pennsylvania, he served under Cutler during the war. He then heeded the professor's call to strengthen the Veterans Adminis-tration, becoming chief at the West Roxbury VA Hospital, orchestrat-ing the first affiliation between a Veterans Hospital and a university, and overseeing a joint surgical training program with the Brigham.

As one of the early surgeons involved in treating vascular disease, Warren was an imaginative and productive clinical investigator. Real-izing that the substitution of abnormal arteries of afflicted patients with the healthy vessels of cadavers was relatively ineffectual despite ongo-ing attempts at preservation and storage, he began to replace aortic aneurysms with synthetic grafts, a long and hazardous operation at the time. While several research groups were testing newly available graft materials, most were generally unsatisfactory. Indeed, one of my tasks as a resident at the West Roxbury VA Hospital was to make aortic tube grafts by sewing together pieces of old nylon spinnaker from his boat.

Warren's expertise in the development of prostheses for amputees was widely recognized. The prevention and treatment of pulmonary emboli, a relatively common problem at the time, also became a major interest. Having examined the benefits of heparin administered subcu-taneously, he turned toward the possibilities of dissolving venous clots in both experimental animals and in patients with thromboembolic disorders.[18] Although he showed that the fibrinolytic agents then available were relatively ineffectual, his work and that of his colleagues in this field presaged by decades the more successful methods now used routinely.[19] The detection of intravascular thrombi using radiolabelled clotting factors was another ongoing interest.

He was widely recognized as the editor of a major journal, the *Archives of Surgery*. In addition to several vascular texts, he edited *Surgery* in collaboration with other members of the Harvard Medical School department of surgery.[20] Modeled in part after Homans's own *Textbook of Surgery*, it was a highly regarded compendium of current concepts and methods. An experienced transatlantic sailor to and from his house in Ireland, he also became an expert in the classification of conifers during his retirement. "All my life I've been interested in diagnosis and things that can go wrong in surgery. This work is no different. It's looking for errors in classification and making pigeonholes, making certain each kind of conifer is in the right pigeonhole and, when it isn't, to be prepared to change."[21]

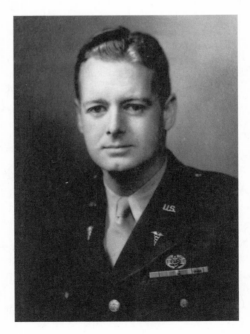

FIGURE 6.5   Chilton Crane.

Chilton Crane spent his entire career at the Brigham. Training under Cutler, he spent nearly three years in the South Pacific during the war, receiving two Bronze Stars. He later described some of his activities. "In the Fall of 1942, because of the vagaries of jungle warfare and the difficulties of transportation through the roots, vines and swamps of the New Guinea Rain Forest, orders came through to set up and supply the Portable Surgical Hospitals [conceptualized and developed by Cutler and Zollinger in Europe]. These small, relatively mobile units were designed and equipped to carry out major surgery in perimeter tents a few hundred feet behind the front lines. Each consisted of four officers and 33 men, the latter including 12 or 14 surgical and medical technicians. Supplies would be carried from landing craft to beach and as far inland as newly bulldozed tracks would allow. Just before embarkation, Dr. Frederick Ross [another of Cutler's trainees who later guided generations of Brigham residents during their surgical rotation at the Burbank Hospital in Fitchburg] took a quick course in urgent dentistry with the view of limiting his shipboard practice to emergency extractions only. Stationed close to the front, these units saved many lives and limbs of the U.S. soldiers involved, by the prompt debridement of innumerable peripheral gunshot, grenade and mortar wounds, and the definitive treatment or drainage of many chest and abdominal wounds. The concept of small, self-contained, relatively mobile units, capable of bringing skilled, fairly definitive surgery close to the front lines in terrain prohibitive of easy travel and transport was completely sound. These proved themselves in their huge contribution to the medical and surgical care of the sick and wounded through six jungle campaigns."[22]

Caring for individuals with peripheral vascular disease throughout much of his career, still an emerging field, Crane's careful surgical dissections, gentleness with his patients, and invariably wry humor made him highly popular among the students, interns, and residents. As a young member of the teaching staff and understanding well Homans's prior observations of the relationship between deep vein thrombosis and its complications, he, like Warren, developed an enduring interest in methods to prevent pulmonary embolism. Using a heparin-gelatin-dextrose mixture (DPO-heparin) as a sole anticoagulant, he treated large numbers of patients with venous thromboembolic disease including those with pulmonary embolism.[23] The majority achieved good results.[24]

As evidence mounted that most major emboli formed in the veins of the calf, surgeons began increasingly to ligate the superficial femoral veins of both legs in patients at risk, as Homans had proposed years before. Indeed, this became one of the most common surgical operations in many hospitals during the 1950s and 1960s despite a failure rate of ten percent and a mortality rate of five percent. In a continuing analysis of clinical data, Crane established general guidelines for venous interruption either at the level of the femoral vein or at the inferior vena cava to control clots migrating from the legs or forming in pelvic veins after an operation.[25] For a time, this rather extreme treatment was performed relatively routinely in patients with mitral valve disease who continued to develop pulmonary emboli regardless of anticoagulation. These extremely ill individuals who filled the hospital beds would arrive from the medical service for operation, invariably sitting up in bed to breathe more easily. Under Crane's guidance, we residents became adept at ligating their inferior vena cava, often under local anesthesia.

As recovery room facilities were inadequate and post-operative monitoring techniques rudimentary, the patients returned directly to the medical wards. Within a few hours after occlusion of their great abdominal vein, many went into shock, stopped excreting urine, and died. Several of us involved with these patients carried out rather extensive studies to understand the then unrecognized alterations in venous circulation which led to apparently massive fluid shifts.[26] Following variations in venous pressure, assessing changes in blood and plasma volume using newly available dye dilution methods, and determining various facets of renal function, we confirmed the obvious: that blood pooling in the legs and pelvis substantially reduced venous return to the heart. The high pressure below the ligature caused significant leakage of fluid and protein through the walls of the distended vessels into the tissues. Hypotension resulted.

The procedure was so morbid that an external clip to narrow the lumen of the vein soon became available to replace the ligature technique. This device allowed adequate blood flow but prevented the migration of clots. A far less invasive internal filter introduced via the jugular vein, in turn, replaced this operative maneuver. The vena caval "umbrella" is used routinely in the prevention of pulmonary embolus in patients unresponsive to anticoagulation.

Warren and Crane included the treatment of pulmonary emboli in their widening vascular interests. A dreaded complication of deep venous thrombosis, pulmonary embolism may produce a rapid catastrophic series of events that often lead to sudden death. The possibility that massive, life-threatening clots could be removed surgically from the lung had been considered for years. In 1908, the German surgeon Frederich Trendelenberg first suggested direct operative intervention, performing the procedure successfully on a calf, then on three patients. Two of these survived 16 and 37 hours postoperatively. In an address to the New England Heart Association in 1933, Cutler had urged that pulmonary embolectomy should be attempted, decrying the currently accepted antipathy against aggressive surgical intervention. "I see no reason why the modern surgeon should not operate, or at least expose the pulmonary artery, on early provocation rather than wait until a fatality is almost certain. A few negative explorations should do no harm and the successful cases that will come under such circumstances, will prove more numerous."[27] Within months, a German surgeon performed the first successful pulmonary embolectomy with survival of the patient.

Regardless of this single success, the majority of surgeons in the United States disagreed with Cutler because of continuing discouragement surrounding the occasional failed attempts and the promise of potentially more effective anticoagulant drugs. A respected academic leader summarized this prevailing opinion at a conference in 1944. "I hope we will not have any more papers on the removal of pulmonary emboli from this organization [American Surgical Association], an operation which should be of historic interest only. Certainly the way to prevent death from pulmonary embolism is to prevent the clot from becoming detached and getting into the pulmonary artery if thrombosis does occur."[28] Unfortunately, prevention of the condition with anticoagulants never completely fulfilled expectations and patients continued to die. But by 1952, 11 additional reports of clot removal had been added to the European literature.

In 1958, Warren and his colleagues performed the first successful pulmonary embolectomy in the United States. The patient was a 65-year-old woman who sustained a massive pulmonary embolus following gall bladder surgery. The authors recommended, as had Cutler a quarter century before that "all patients in whom the diagnosis is suspected be taken to the operating room where, rather than on the ward, the diagnostic steps should be undertaken and the final decision for or against surgery be made. When the diagnosis is sure, and the embolus is of a size to cause sustained circulatory embarrassment, operation should be undertaken without waiting for the agonal phase. Modern experience with the management of cardiac arrest and resuscitation was responsible for the survival of this patient and should be used to advantage in others. The addition of interruption of major veins to prevent further embolism is a feature of the management which should not be neglected."[29] The way had been opened for increasing application and success for this type of heroic venture. With better radiologic diagnosis and the availability of cardiopulmonary bypass, pulmonary embolectomy has been lifesaving in many patients.

CHAPTER 7

CARL WALTER, SURGICAL ENGINEERING, AND THE TEACHING OF THE CRAFT

FROM AMONG THE legacies of Cutler's highly regarded trainees, the contributions of Carl Walter have remained critical to operative and peri-operative care to this day. A colorful and enduring figure during his four decades at the Brigham, a professor of surgery and practicing surgeon, Walter held many medical patents, founded and directed a renowned biomedical company, pioneered advances in blood transfusions and hospital engineering, and was a seminal figure in improving aseptic technique and control of infections in surgical patients. His extensive orange groves in Florida were highly productive. A successful fundraiser at Harvard Medical School, he endowed two academic chairs. Today, students and faculty attend lectures in the Walter Auditorium.

But despite his plethora of accomplishments, he was perhaps unappreciated by many of the residency staff, as his presence on the wards was relatively infrequent and the significance of his advances not directly obvious. Aloof to those who did not know him, he often appeared as an outspoken and authoritarian figure. Many of his peers thought he had been trained as an engineer before entering medical school because of his expertise in a variety of clinically relevant disciplines that encompassed blood banking, autoclaves, and the hemodialysis machine. Although this was not the case, his early summer jobs may have kindled a later interest in technology and its applications to patient care and safety.

He initially worked at a construction site. "I spent all my time in the summer either lugging beer to the workmen or picking up nails, always watching what was going on. It was a liberal education. [I] learned all about plumbing. Of course, there was no electricity then. It was all gas pipes." He accrued additional practical experience with the telephone company. "My only engineering background, if you want to call it that, was in high school in Cleveland. I worked as a lineman for [the telephone company] during vacations. They gave us a hell of a good course in electricity. I was involved in work with cables, man-holes, and installations. The clips [on the wires] were put on and taken off several times. I had been wearing the leg irons all day, and got tired, so I took my safety strap and hooked it to the cable and sat in it as a hammock as I worked. I didn't get the clips off fast enough. The [phone line] had a 500 volt circuit. Zap! Off I went flying from the pole, across the alley, and onto a tin roof. When I got up I said, 'to hell with this. If this is what life is all about, I quit.' I did, and went back to school."[1]

As he had compiled good grades and was a fast quarter miler on his high school track team, the Harvard Club of Cleveland arranged that he receive a scholarship to Harvard College. By chance, Elliott Cutler was chairman of the committee. Subsequent periodic reports and meetings between the two men during vacations created a close and durable relationship. "At the end of my senior year he asked, 'What are you going to do?' I said 'I got a job with Dupont. I am going to be a chemist in the research department.' He said 'Carl don't waste your time on the nuts and bolts of chemistry; you ought to get working with people; you ought to go to medical school.' I answered: 'I can't do that. I'm broke and it's too late to be admitted.' 'Well, we will fix that.' He promptly telephoned someone I later learned to respect a great deal, the Assistant Dean of Harvard Medical School. Cutler introduced me, I got quizzed long distance and two minutes later he said, 'You are admitted.' So I turned to Cutler: 'That's easy enough to say but I've got no money, so I can't go to medical school. I have got to go to work and pay off my college debt.' 'I'll fix that.' he said. He called a shipping magnate in Cleveland. He explained the situation, and I got a loan for my education—bang—just like that."[2]

Walter's expertise in chemistry came to fruition during medical school when he developed a micromethod for blood analysis. Indeed, he supported himself at night by carrying out blood chemistry deter-minations on patients at the New England Baptist Hospital. He joined the Brigham surgical house staff in 1933, falling quickly under the influence of Robert Zollinger. The chief resident became an important supporter and protector of his increasingly iconoclastic intern, often taking his side against the hospital administration, as he did during the incident of the blue water. "At that time, the house officer initiate gathered specimens, did the laboratory work, recorded results, started intravenous infusions, inserted hypodermic needles, encoded diagnoses, assisted at transfusions, selected instruments, and served as [the] instrument man during operations. Occasionally, he was drafted to hold a retractor. Pupship chores bored me because I had operated an active clinical laboratory while a medical student. Fortunately, however, the scut work exposed me to challenging hazards of hospitalization that spurred my interest and usurped my time. Conflicts with the resident about where I spent my time promptly arose. Soon these were aggravated by hostility on the part of the hospital officialdom that personalized the demonstration of the hazards. Zollie promptly identified with this pup and provided such an effective umbrella that I was able to successfully survive the house officership while also investigating sanitary plumbing, the preparation of safe parenteral fluid, creation of a blood bank, and developing effective sterilization practices. These by-products of our association would prove to have a lasting impact on surgery."[3]

Walter wanted to become a neurosurgeon. Cutler, however, impressed with his abilities to solve puzzles and repair defects in hospital design and epidemiology, kept distracting him with relevant projects until the time to apply had run out. "The challenges to improve surgical care at the Brigham during my term as House Officer, demonstrate how serendipity can broaden a career. My attention and time were diverted from the drill and chain-gang-like duties of internship by shockingly anachronistic techniques. I rediscovered principles of patient care established decades earlier as I divided my time between learning the art and practice of surgery and improving the technical care of surgical patients."[4]

Improving the technical care of surgical patients took several forms. Walter developed an enduring interest in the causes of surgical sepsis soon after he began his internship.[5] The severe pyrogenic reactions with chills and fever that often developed in patients who had received intravenous fluid therapy created such a furor that Henry Christian forbad the use of parenteral fluids by his house staff. Because of his concerns, only surgical residents were allowed to give such treatment to the dehydrated patients on the medical service. Christian's medical residents bypassed this ruling by transferring the sick individuals to surgery for rehydration then transferring them immediately back to their own units.

While Cushing himself had investigated the effects of electrolyte solutions and had considered their intravenous administration years before, his interest had lapsed in part because of unfortunate experiences with a poorly performing sterilizer. Hearing about Walter's efforts, he admitted in a letter to Cutler in 1935: "As a matter of fact, in the early years of the hospital, being uneasy about the sterility of the fluids, I ceased using them for intravenous therapy. I am glad you have put someone to work on the subject, for it is high time it was reviewed."[6] Cutler agreed and assigned his intern to "do something to put parenteral therapy on a sound footing." Walter began to examine the existing methods. He later described the progression of events.

"At that time, Cushing's solution was formulated at each nursing unit by adding the contents of a powder pack, compounded individually in the hospital pharmacy, to a liter of boiling distilled water. The [cooled] solution was poured into a buret and administered [to the patient] through used rubber tubing and a glass adapter affixed to a needle. The glass burets were stained and often opaque and sticky.

"My investigations of the cause of the chills, fever and shock-like state was first undertaken in a corner of the laboratory being abandoned by Harvey Cushing as he retired to Yale. To me, as an enthusiastic chemist, safe parenteral fluids meant chemical purity. Efforts were mounted to clean glassware, tubing, connectors and needles as these would be readied for quantitative chemical analysis. The assembled apparatus was sterilized by steam. Nonetheless, severe reactions persisted. I applied [a new] rabbit technique to test the parenteral fluids and promptly identified endotoxins in both the distilled water and the dry chemical constituents. Distilled water was dispensed by the pharmacy in glass flasks plugged with a gauze sponge tied neatly in place. Although intended to be used promptly, the flask often stood for days prior to use. Sometimes a fine white sediment accumulated which was shown to be of silica as well as various bacteria. Muddy water, an accumulation of years, was found in the evaporator of the pharmacy still.

"To obviate these problems, I designed a reflux type of still that produced steam from running water. A Pyrex glass prototype with tapered neck then a full-scale metal version [were later perfected and produced commercially]. These provided an endless supply of particulate free distilled water that passed the rabbit test repeatedly over months without the burdensome maintenance required by conventional stills. I administered the fluids processed by the new technique to consecutive patients without an untoward reaction following any of 1000 infusions. Parenteral therapy was rapidly accepted throughout the hospital and dehydrated medical patients were no longer surreptitiously transferred by the resident staff to surgical wards at night for hydration. A direct steam jacketed sterilizer was installed in a corridor outside Cushing's laboratory. Soon, operating room supplies were being processed. Within a year the makeshift operation gave way to a new concept—a central supply room for the entire hospital."[7]

Walter's success with parenteral infusion provoked an interest in the subject of sterilizers. These devices were rudimentary in the 1930s and, as he relates, often remarkably ineffectual. "Elliott Cutler noticed that a lot of herniorrophies ended up disrupting and draining before healing. They developed a puffiness and crepitation, a sort of low grade gas gangrene. The patients had mild fever. My first five herniorrophies had it. We traced it back to a cancer of the sigmoid that John Homans had done. The instruments supposedly had been sterilized and then recirculated. We cultured anaerobes from the instruments first and then from the sterilizer, both before and after so-called sterilization. But the instruments and the sterilizer were all unsterile! It was a big eye opener to me that although everything was unsterile, so few people got into trouble. That was how I discovered that the steam sterilizers don't sterilize."[8]

In fact, not only didn't the sterilizers sterilize, but the ice cubes Walter placed in the back of the horizontal autoclave cylinder did not melt despite correct setting of temperature, time, and cycle. Steam circulated around the front of the space particularly toward the top, but never made it to the lower back corners. He also noted that the location of the thermostat beyond the check valve in the sterilizer gave readings that had little relevance to the actual temperature within the apparatus. The manufacturers took such umbrage to the adverse publicity directed toward their product following his presentation of his findings to a surgical audience at a major conference, that they generated two angry lawsuits, ultimately dropped. He quickly corrected the deficits of the existing system and built a vertical autoclave to clean and sterilize the bloody, oily instruments. The entire process of cleansing

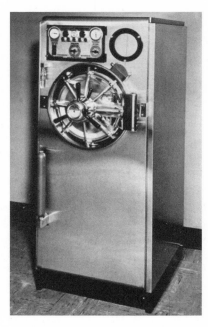

FIGURE 7.1   One of Carl Walter's sterilizers. This one was in continuous use in the Surgical Research Laboratory at Harvard Medical School for over 50 years.

with detergent then steam exposure only took a few minutes. This concept led to the creation of a reliable technique of "flash sterilization" that he reported several years later.

His knowledge of the workings of these machines never wavered. I approached him years later in hopes of a donation toward a new sterilizer to replace the one which had been in the Surgical Research Laboratory for nearly four decades. We used this apparatus daily to sterilize the instruments for the ongoing experiments and weekly to prepare for the student dog course. The problem, as I explained to him, was that the sterilizer could no longer mount appropriate steam pressure. He came over to the lab, examined the elderly structure carefully and found, deeply hidden in the back, a kinked intake pipe. Straightening it within moments, he pronounced the unit healthy. And healthy it remained, functioning well for two additional decades.

He sharpened his latent interest in thermostat mechanics a few years later by serendipity during a research project when he attempted to control the temperature of an aquarium in which swam Golden Moon tropical fish. These fish developed melanomas when the water was kept slightly warm. A constant ambient temperature was difficult to maintain, however, because of the inadequacy of the existing thermostats. Discussion of the problem led to a collaboration with an acquaintance who had developed a promising device. After refining the apparatus to control accurately the aquarium temperature, all the fish grew melanomas. Indeed, the thermostats became so highly regarded that they were used successfully in the engines of Spitfire airplanes during World War II and are still placed in many commercial jet engines throughout the world. The two investigators then joined Thomas Fenn, an enthusiastic financial backer and one of Walter's neighbors, to form the company *Fenwal*, to which Fenn and Walter lent their names. Increasingly involved in the production of high precision devices and blood bank technology, it eventually opened plants in England, France, Italy, and Japan.

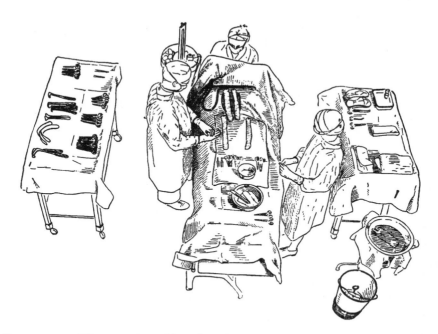

Figure 7.2   The operating table and scrub table arranged for surgery. From Walter CW, *The Aseptic Treatment of Wounds* (New York: Macmillan, 1948), 54.

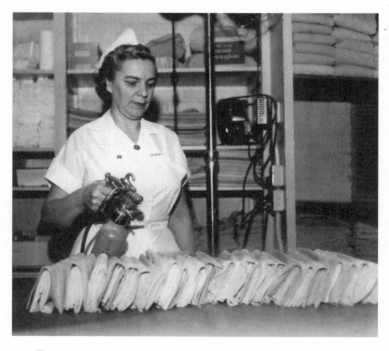

FIGURE 7.3   Brigham nurse sterilizing packed rubber gloves.

Walter's uncompromising efforts to improve hospital safety and standardize routine activities and efficiencies in the operating room often flew in the face of already accepted protocols. His concern with multiple facets of the care of surgical patients culminated in a widely respected text, *Aseptic Treatment of Wounds*.[9] A vade mecum placed in every operating room in the country and revered by generations of nurses and young surgeons, its principles did much to increase safety during surgery. Appropriately, he borrowed the title from the classic paper on the subject that Lord Lister had published 80 years before. Not only did he discuss in the text methods to sterilize instruments and the importance of circulating the air surrounding the patient, he described in detail virtually all of the maneuvers taken for granted in the modern operating room. These ranged from the most effective techniques of scrubbing the hands and proper cleansing of the operative site, to efficient organization of instruments and linens on the operating table. These practices are used to this day.

In addition to these substantial contributions, Walter was responsible for much of modern blood banking technology. Occasional transfusions between animals, animals and man, and between humans had been carried out in the seventeenth and eighteenth centuries. All were unsuccessful. While the identification of blood groups by Ernst Landsteiner in Vienna in 1900 allowed appropriate matching between individuals, the use of stored blood for transfusions did not become possible until the discovery that the addition of small amounts of sodium citrate could prevent clotting outside the body. But despite these advances, techniques to transfuse blood safely and consistently remained rudimentary for decades. In his 1931 *Textbook of Surgery*, John Homans summarized the existing situation that Walter faced as a house officer and that the clinical surgeons of the time had to consider before undertaking complex surgical procedures. Many of these conditions existed until after World War II.

"The present day methods of transfusion represent the culmination of attempts, dating back many centuries, to introduce the blood of healthy persons into the veins of the sick. Modern blood transfusion began as a direct union of an artery of the donor with a vein of the recipient. The technique was difficult, the dosage of blood was utterly uncertain, and the vessels of both donor and recipient were sacrificed. To overcome the technical difficulty of uniting artery to vein or vein to vein, mechanical devices were invented. But it was not until methods were devised by which a known quantity of blood could be drawn from a *vein* of one individual and, in the same completely aseptic and fluid state, injected into another, that blood transfusion came into common use. To accomplish this object there are now available at least four methods; the sodium citrate method, the syringe cannula method, the stop-cock method, and the paraffin-coated tube method. Since the technique of blood transfusion is certain to undergo further modification, it is enough to say that each embodies a different scheme for the prevention of coagulation or deterioration of fresh blood in transit from the vein of donor to the recipient. All four methods may to some extent injure the red corpuscles of the donor, and it is to the by-products of this injury that the thermal reactions and chills after transfusion are probably due."[10]

With these less-than-appealing choices, the obvious need for better techniques for blood replacement crystallized in Walter's mind following a "spectacular misadventure" that occurred while he was a fourth-year medical student in 1932. "I became party to an emergency transfusion essential for supporting the patient following a massive hemorrhage Harvey Cushing encountered during enucleation of a meningioma. A compatible donor was brought into the operating room on a stretcher. The inside of a long buret with a "s" shaped stem [part of the transfusion apparatus] had to be coated with paraffin to delay clotting of the blood it would collect. My assignment was to warm the buret over an alcohol lamp and to keep rotating it while melted paraffin was introduced in an attempt to achieve an even coating. Finally, a stopper with an integral suction bulb was inserted and sealed in place. The stem was inserted into an incised phlebotomy at the donor's elbow. Suction was applied and the blood was slowly sucked into the buret. On this particular occasion, the anesthetist demanded a faster transfusion; greater suction was applied and suddenly, the buret imploded with a tremendous spattering of blood. 'J . . . C . . .' I explained, 'there must be a better way.' Dr. Cushing quietly commanded: 'Whoever said that, come to my office after surgery.' When I arrived, he was furious that anyone would curse in his operating room. I had to admit that I did not know of a better technique for transfusion. His command, 'Well, you had best find one' inspired my lifelong interest in techniques for collection, storage and transfusion of blood and in no small way shaped one facet of my career."[11]

Problems with red cell lysis and bacterial contamination were always present. Reports of a relatively successful blood storage operation carried out at a casualty clearing station in France during World War I piqued Walter's fancy, particularly as he realized that many of the techniques he had developed for safe parenteral fluids could be adapted to blood banking. However, as the Brigham Hospital Trustees considered dealing in blood "immoral and unethical," the blood bank was a secret operation housed beneath Cushing's surgical artist's in the studio basement. They soon appreciated the importance of its services, however, and granted space upstairs. The operation soon spread to nearby hospitals, as well as providing blood products to laboratories in the medical school. Indeed, for years, Walter was the only person in the hospital allowed to transfuse patients. His solo role included typing, cross matching and storage. He also founded the Red Cross Blood Bank in Boston during World War II, collecting 84,000 units. The devices he created during this period to separate red blood cells from plasma, and albumin from other protein components are still used.

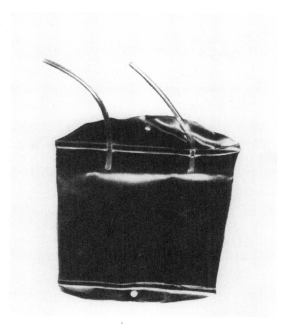

Figure 7.4   The plastic blood bag.

But adequate preservation of blood remained a critical unsolved problem, as it was stored routinely but often ineffectually in glass bottles with rubber stoppers. Its subsequent administration through reusable rubber tubing was cumbersome and provided ingress for bacteria. By the Thanksgiving recess in 1947, however, Walter had produced a hermetically sealed, hemorepellent and durable plastic blood bag with the donor tubing and administration ports integrated into the completely closed system. This was a significant contribution to the new field of blood banking. He describes the evolving events. "I fashioned hot wire potents to join the parts of the system—bag, donor tube, and delivery ports. The following Monday, my patent council was elated and the patent application was drafted—one of the eventual 37. The prototype bags worked well with water or with outdated blood. The compressible compliant bags could be filled and emptied by gravity and withstood centrifugation. Plasma could be extracted and the formed elements separated. Pressure infusion could be done."[12]

He presented his bag in 1949 to those attending a conference on the preservation of blood held at the medical school and sponsored jointly by the National Institutes of Health, the American Red Cross and the National Research Council. The audience was entranced. One participant described the occasion. "It was at that time and in connection with that conference that I first came to know Carl Walter. Until then blood was collected through rubber tubing into glass bottles, and it was already appreciated that important elements of the blood were damaged or altered during the collection process. It was against that backdrop that Carl came over one day to a meeting of the planning group and produced a plastic bag, fully distended with blood, which he then casually dropped on the floor and stood upon. We are so accustomed now to these plastic bags, not only for blood, but for all kinds of other fluids, that it is difficult to appreciate the enormous impact that Carl Walter's bag had on the United States health care system."[13]

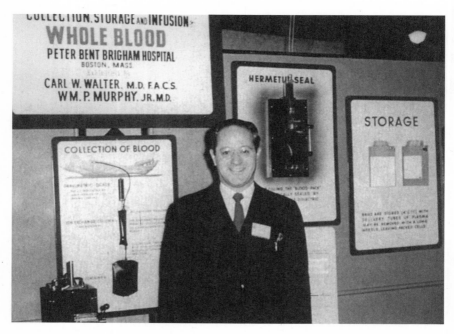

Figure 7.5   Walter presenting his blood banking techniques at the American College of Surgeons meeting in 1948.

But despite the excellence of the new blood bag, difficulties remained. Bags of plasma fractured when frozen. The bags containing anticoagulant burst during sterilization. Worse—fungi grew in the "sterilized" plastic itself within a week on the shelf. He and his co-workers ultimately solved these problems by switching to a plasticized polyvinyl chloride material for the bag, designing and patenting a sterilizer for the flexible blood containers, and mixing air and steam to allow more sterilizing energy. At the same time, they produced a stainless steel donor needle with a hemorepellant interior surface and a tamperproof cover, the only piece of equipment separate from the closed plastic system.

The improved blood bags were used extensively and effectively during the Korean War and have been in universal use since in all blood banks. As most commercial firms were not interested initially in these innovations, Walter and his co-workers used the facilities at *Fenwal*. While the technology was a complete system change from existing techniques, like many of Walter's other inventions, it was a major innovation in patient care. Fenwal was eventually sold to the *Baxter-Travenol Company*.

THE SURGICAL RESEARCH LABORATORY was an abiding feature of the department of surgery throughout the existence of the Peter Bent Brigham and during the first decades of the Brigham and Women's. The advances produced by investigators working there over the nearly ninety years of its existence have meant much to the entire field of surgery and to student and post-graduate education. When Cutler became chief, he continued Cushing's long-established tradition of inviting his best residents to spend time in research as Arthur Tracy Cabot Fellows before returning to the wards. Cushing had stressed that the experience they received was critical to their future careers. "The responsibility thrown on a young man early in his career of 'running a laboratory' where both teaching and research are actually engaged in with the least possible supervision and interference on the part of his seniors, is a character making episode."[14] Cutler agreed. "The influence of our surgical laboratory in the Medical School on the overall professional thinking and care of the patients has always been a large one. Here, problems arising in their clinic have been tested for their value, and here also technical problems have reached solutions before human attempts have been made. A considerable amount of the professional credit accruing to this hospital has come from work done in the Laboratory for Surgical Research. The men trained here as Arthur Tracy Fellows, almost without exception, have obtained high positions."[15]

As may occur in all laboratories hosting individuals aspiring to remain in an academic setting, the results of this long-term philosophy varied. Zollinger later expanded on the theme, perhaps somewhat more realistically than his professors. "For a resident with [academic] aspirations to be invited to go to the dog lab for a year was a signal to that individual and his co-workers that the Chief had selected him as potential future chief resident. Other residents tended to finish their training sooner and go out into practice or into a specialty. During this year the resident assigned to the lab was really the responsible man for its direction. He either did well or else! Animals were cheap and I don't recall that expense or the need for a 'grant' was ever considered! Many of us carried out major gastrointestinal procedures simply to improve our technical skills."[16]

But despite many young surgeons simply improving their technical skills, a few inevitably became dedicated to basic and applied research and drove their fields of interest forward during their subsequent careers. Much of their enthusiasm depended upon the interest and guidance of the professor. The early contributions of Weed, Goetsch, Holman, and others were original and important. In the main, however, basic investigative output under Cushing remained relatively static. For him, the laboratory and the operating room were one; reports of studies based upon patients, their diseases, and their surgical treatment poured from his pen.

Laboratory activity increased during Cutler's tenure, although the majority of the projects involved refining and practicing operative techniques (such as Zollinger's "major gastrointestinal procedures") more than novel physiologic investigations. But there were significant exceptions. For instance, in his 1939 report to Cutler on projects ongoing in the laboratory, Dunphy, a productive young investigator at the time, summarized his own interests. These included studies of wound healing, shock, transplantation of the adrenal gland, attempts at arteriovenous fistulae, and x-ray treatment of peritonitis. As the Cabot Fellow and titular head of the laboratory, he also reviewed the ongoing efforts of his laboratory colleagues. Robert Gross was examining physiological changes in dogs after production and closure of an artificial ductus arteriosus. Harrison was investigating renal ischemia, and Walter was continuing his studies on sterilization and surgical asepsis. Some of these early projects blossomed into lifelong objects of concentration.

With a modern ring, Dunphy described the laboratory personnel and decried the lack of funds: "This past year has been a very pleasant and harmonious one as far as the laboratory is concerned. The present laboratory staff is very well trained and competent. Mel [a technician], however, is getting old, and sooner or later it will be necessary to change. Possibly this winter it will be necessary for him to work half-time and some boy should be broken in. Roy [another technician] is an unusually bright, capable, and willing worker. We are fortunate to have him and should make every effort to keep him. He is underpaid and certainly cannot afford to continue working with us at his present salary. If the laboratory cannot afford to pay him more, I think his future lies in getting work elsewhere. I have encouraged him to do this. If he continues with the laboratory he deserves more money than he is getting."[17]

Much of the credit for the laboratory work under Cutler's aegis must go to Carl Walter (a Cabot Fellow himself), who served as overall laboratory director between 1937 and 1949 and educated a panoply of talented students, residents and research workers.[18] As Cutler himself noted "Walter acts as a mentor to Arthur Tracy Cabot Fellows by continuing his work in the laboratory and making the laboratory his professional home. His unusual abilities have led to his developing and perfecting certain tangible methods of great benefit to surgeons."[19] During his directorship and for years thereafter, the laboratory was an important nidus for communication between investigators and clinicians. For instance, the tradition of laboratory conferences flourished, usually in conjunction with lunch or tea. These meetings included "speakers both from our group and elsewhere. The opportunity for interchange of ideas between laboratory and clinic and between physicians and surgeons, between visitor and native is a much needed leaven for the weeks work."[20] Cutler often presided.

Dunphy later confirmed these sentiments in a letter. "During my stay in the laboratory, I was greatly influenced by Carl Walter. His critical sense regarding the running of the laboratory, the care of animals, the handling of technicians, and the nature of truly sound scientific inquiry were passed on to me in a way that I have appreciated since. I really believe that [his] influence on all of us who worked in the laboratory in those days was one of the most valuable aspects of our entire experience. One thing was certain. Carl Walter knew the lab and although he was no longer its immediate director, he kept in touch with everything that was going on. He was the first to recognize incompetent, inaccurate, or unreliable work. A great many people never understood him because of his frank and direct approach, but I would like to put a plug in for him in any account of the surgical laboratory in those days. I can honestly say that I learned more about physiology, physiological research, and investigation in general from Carl Walter than from many others with whom I worked before or since."[21]

Despite the avowed intention of Cutler to give the Cabot Fellow full autonomy in the laboratory, a certain petulance showed up sporadically throughout Dunphy's report as to the real person in charge. "As long as Dr. Walter maintains an office in the laboratory and is nominally the director of the laboratory, there will be a conflict between him and the ATC Fellow unless there is a precise understanding of their relative functions in running the laboratory. There is no doubt that Dr. Walter knows more about the laboratory than the last three ATC Fellows put together. This is only logical because he has been there three times as long. It is impossible for any boy to come to the laboratory and immediately take control without mistakes which inevitably will bring about a conflict. Moreover, it is unfair to the Fellow to give him the impression that he is in full charge of the laboratory, when, in point of fact, he isn't." However, Dunphy concluded that all was well. "It can be said that the laboratory runs smoothly and efficiently. Dr. [Richard] Warren could hardly believe that a laboratory could run as satisfactorily as ours after his recent experiences in Philadelphia."

THE COURSE IN ASEPTIC TECHNIQUE was an important responsibility of the Surgical Research Laboratory during Cutler's tenure. Because of its high profile and success in the curriculum at Harvard Medical School, similar courses arose in other teaching hospitals in Boston then disseminated to many medical schools throughout the country. The students carried out surgical exercises on dogs that mimicked as closely as possible actual operations performed on patients. They organized and packed supplies, selected and sterilized instruments, administered anesthesia, performed the operations, made rounds on the animal ward postoperatively, and undertook a postmortem examination if necessary. The instructors emphasized keeping an ether chart and writing accurate notes and records. This experience for the students was also important in recruiting them into surgery.

Walter oversaw the course for many years. Besides being an excellent teacher, he is remembered as an exacting taskmaster. If a surgical resident or a medical student was bending too much over the operative field, he could expect a sharp blow on his back from the instructor, coupled with appropriate opprobrium. He taught the students to scrub properly by covering their hands with lamp black then blindfolding them. The challenge then came to get their hands clean. Despite their best efforts, he sent them back to the sink again and again. Finally, after scrubbing was completed, Walter would drop a quarter on the floor before the student and strongly comment on the victim's instinctive retrieval of the coin. However, such lessons learned were not forgotten, and surgeons to this day remember his training maneuvers with wry amusement and great appreciation. Indeed, his involvement in the surgical course and in the organization

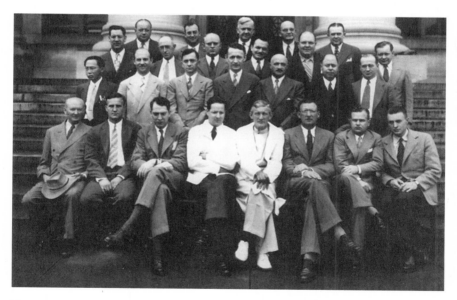

FIGURE 7.6 Cutler's course in surgical technique given for community surgeons during World War II.

of the Surgical Research Laboratory stimulated the development and improvement of multiple techniques for asepsis in the operating room, familiarity with surgical procedures, and details of postoperative care. They were of lasting benefit to clinical surgery.

The scope of the instruction broadened during the 1930s and 1940s when Cutler and Zollinger, then Walter, offered extensive teaching sessions on technique and new innovations to graduate students and community surgeons. The effort became especially important during the years of involvement of the United States in World War II when many members of the surgical staff were abroad. Indeed, at the suggestion of the Army Medical Corps, the dog course increased in size to provide in many cases the only surgical training young men obtained before joining the conflict.

His efforts and those of his instructors were so successful that Francis Newton, acting for a time as surgeon-in-chief during Cutler's absence in the European Theater, appeared sometimes overwhelmed by the extent of the teaching load. "During the war, many former students wrote letters of appreciation from isolated corners of the world when they found themselves forced to do surgery with little training other than that received in the laboratory. It of interest to examine the situation in which the surgical service of the Brigham finds itself today (1945) as compared to 1941. We have today 18 teachers available (above intern grade) to carry the entire teaching program on a year round accelerated basis, as opposed to 30 in 1941. The subtraction has been natural in that group who are fit for military service—youthful, enthusiastic, well-trained men. And yet, the number of teaching hours and the numbers of students to teach has increased in the following way: In the 12 months of 1941, 48 students took the second year course in operating room technique. In 1944 there were 124. Ninety in 1941 took the third year course in surgical techniques; 187 took the same course in 1944."[22]

This focus on operative technique sharpened by the demands of the war had an unexpected result. The course attracted qualified surgeons who wanted to improve their abilities. But within a year or two general practitioners and "various-fly-by-nights and n'er-do-wells" applied to "learn how to do surgery like out of a cook book."[23] Indeed, when this type of instruction came to an end, all involved with the teaching were much relieved because they had, as Francis Moore further commented, "a hand in training a lot of unqualified surgeons to do surgical operations much as a monkey can be taught to run a typewriter. I have never elaborated on this idea for reasons that are quite obvious!" Zollinger remarked that the exercise may have had its uses as "some of our so-called 'two week graduates' did pretty well as they returned home [from the war]. Some of the funds from their tuition were used to pay the secretary for post-graduate studies in the dean's office as well as supplies in the surgical laboratory."[24] Dunphy added: "Most of us felt it was a dramatic, but perhaps a not very appropriate post-graduate exercise! I suspect the best that came out of it were some patient referrals to Cutler and Zollinger."

Despite this modest disenchantment, the course remained popular and continued virtually unchanged until the 1980s. Moore later summarized its aims. "The laboratory contributes to the education of the medical students by courses in surgical technique given to the second and third year classes. Early in the second year, a three hour demonstration, culminating in a laparotomy on a dog, is intended to give a panoramic view of the preparation of supplies, care of instruments, sterilization, disinfection of the skin, aseptic operating room technique, the rudiments of surgical technique, and terminal sterilization of some of the equipment. Groups of students then carry out themselves what they have seen demonstrated. Five exercises are held in which each student performs a surgical procedure on an anesthetized dog, including giving the ether anesthesia. Third year students are given a series of 12 exercises in full surgical technique, including anesthesia and asepsis. Thus, the student develops a modest proficiency in handling instruments and ligatures, hemostasis and suturing."[25]

Overall, the course in aseptic technique was a wonderful exercise. John Rowbotham, one of Moore's early residents and a surgeon at the Deaconess Hospital, and I taught it for years before it was discontinued because of rapidly increasing costs to the department. My wife, Mary Graves Tilney, was supervisor of the laboratory for nearly three decades. It fell to her to order the dogs during the 6-week course, organize the supplies and make sure all equipment was in place for up to 15 tables. At least 50 medical students attended each year. We still occasionally meet individuals who tell us that the course was the high point of their medical school curriculum and was the reason that they entered surgery.

CHAPTER 8

Surgery of the Heart

The correction of mechanical defects of the heart was an enduring interest for surgeons at the Peter Bent Brigham. Cushing's investigations at Johns Hopkins on the creation of lesions of the cardiac valves were a preamble to Cutler's own efforts, while the later contributions of Charles Hufnagel and Robert Gross, Dwight Harken, John Collins, Lawrence Cohn, and others advanced the field substantially.

Despite the long-established antipathy of surgeons toward operating on the heart or even considering such a step, it is intriguing that in 1908 Cushing published a detailed paper from the Hunterian Laboratories in which he reported the production of abnormalities of cardiac valves in dogs. "In November, 1905, there was brought to the laboratory a large Newfoundland dog suffering with general anasarca, ascites, and other sequelae of passive congestion due to tricuspid insufficiency with compensatory failure resulting from advanced chronic endocarditis. Autopsy disclosed a thickened mitral valve, a dilated and hypertrophied heart showing tricuspid insufficiency, together with an unusually marked degree of venous congestion. Being then unaware that bloody ascites could result from chronic passive congestion of cardiac origin, we undertook to reproduce this condition experimentally. It was necessary, for the success of the investigation, that the animal should survive a sufficient time for the late consequence of the valvular lesions to manifest themselves."[1]

The student course in pathologic physiology that Cushing had organized for the Johns Hopkins medical students heightened his enthusiasm for investigating changes in cardiac function. The pathologist in charge, W.G. MacCallum, emphasized that disorders of organ systems should be taught not only from a morphological standpoint but also in a dynamic form. "It was planned to produce experimentally

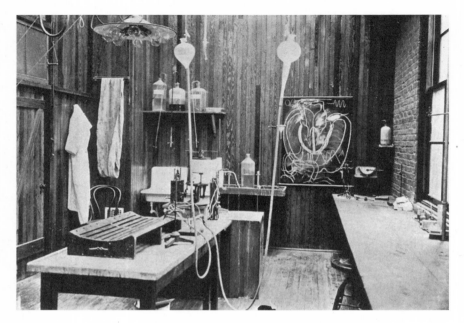

FIGURE 8.1   Cushing's cardiac surgical laboratory at Hopkins, 1908.

such lesions in the various organs as are commonly met with in the wards and any available methods were used to this end."[2] MacCallum and his surgical colleague soon showed that rapid distention of the canine pericardium with fluid increased venous pressure and diminished pulmonary and arterial pressure. Ventricular function declined. The investigators then devised means of producing chronic cardiac valvular lesions to assess their systemic manifestations, creating aortic insufficiency by inserting a blunt probe retrograde down the carotid artery to rupture the valve, and disrupted the mitral or tricuspid valves by introducing a cutting hook through the auricular appendages via an intrathoracic approach.

Experimental means to narrow the heart valves proved more difficult. Cushing and his team created mitral stenosis by partially closing the valvular ring with an external screw clamp or suture, or by passing a strong ligature on a blunt needle through two mitral leaflets or their chordae and tying it tightly in the ventricular cavity. They dipped the ligature into boiling vaseline before its placement to prevent it from becoming a source of thrombus. They even attempted to repair the valve of Jack Gladstone, a 12-year-old English Setter that had arrived in the surgical laboratory on February 28, 1907 with severe ascites. Although they diagnosed mitral stenosis, they were unsuccessful in correcting the defect.

These early attempts to produce valvular lesions were significant for several reasons. The operative approach was unique, "the first exposure of the heart with subsequent recoveries." Indeed, the survival of 11 of 25 animals indicated for the first time that heart valves could be manipulated with some degree of success. It also became clear that the heart muscle could be sutured effectively to control hemorrhage. The respirations of the subjects were sustained when the chest was open by a positive pressure respirator connected to the bronchial tree and lungs via a tracheostomy. Noting that the tracheal defects healed quickly in 35 dogs after removal of the cannulae, Cushing became so confident with the technique that he began to use it immediately in some of his neurosurgical patients who had developed respiratory failure secondary to high intracranial pressure.[3]

As the research group became more adept at operations on the hearts of living dogs, they increasingly considered the possibility that surgical intervention could alleviate the symptoms of patients with severe valvular disease. They were also becoming aware of scattered examples of operations upon the walls of the human heart. There had been 56 such instances by 1904; 40% of the patients recovered. And despite the general disapprobation by many of their peers, a few surgeons were becoming increasingly aware that successful manipulation of the beating heart was possible. The times were ripening for the step between closure of accidental cardiac wounds and entering the chambers to repair valvular abnormalities.

In his publication on the possibilities of heart surgery, Cushing quoted the remarks made in 1903 by Sir Lauder Brunton, a London physician particularly knowledgeable about the effects of drugs on the organ. Brunton had stressed that surgical techniques should be perfected in animals to alleviate mitral stenosis in patients. "Mitral stenosis is not only one of the most distressing forms of cardiac disease, but in its severe forms it resists all treatment by medicine. In looking at the contracted mitral orifice in a severe case of this disease, one is impressed by the hopelessness of ever finding a remedy which will enable the atrium to drive the blood in sufficient stream through the small mitral orifice and the wish unconsciously arises that one could divide the constriction as easily during life as one can after death. The risk which such an operation would entail naturally makes one shrink from it, but in some cases it might be well worthwhile for the patients to balance the risk of a short life against the certainty of a prolonged period of existence which hardly could be called life, and the only conditions under which it could be continued might then be worse than death. But no one would be justified in attempting such a dangerous maneuver as dividing a mitral stenosis on a fellow creature without having first tested its practicality and perfected his technique by previous trials on animals."[4]

Before World War I, Cushing, the neurosurgeon, had refined methods to open the chest and control the respirations, and had shown that animals could recover following operative procedures on the heart either indirectly via adjacent blood vessels or directly through its chambers. Elliott Cutler was well aware of his mentor's experience when he initiated his own forays into heart surgery.

CUTLER BECAME INTERESTED early in his career in the possibilities of surgical relief of significant valvular heart disease. Initial discussions with Samuel Levine, a physician and fellow resident, continued during the research period they both spent at Rockefeller Institute upon their return from Europe after World War I. They were also aware of ongoing studies by other groups. In 1920, for instance, German investigators reported the results of creating valvular insufficiency in animals.[5] Occasionally surgeons had even attempted to open stenotic valves in patients.[6]

Enthused by the existing data and particularly by Brunton's sentiments toward alleviating mitral stenosis in afflicted patients, Cutler, Levine, and resident Claude Beck initiated a series of relevant laboratory experiments to address the condition and its treatment. They studied the effects of transient clamping of the great vessels to and from the hearts of cats and dogs, then began to create valvular stenoses using Cushing's old techniques (ligation and plication of the leaflets) or by holding radium next to the valve edges to form scar.[7] At the same time, they examined a series of human hearts with mitral disease which had been removed at autopsy. Realizing that the heavily calcified valves would be difficult for a small knife to penetrate, they devised a cardiovalvulotome to excise a portion of the involved structure.[8] They produced mitral insufficiency in dogs by inserting the valvulotome through the base of the left ventricle in preference to entering the left auricular appendage with the attendant risks of dislodging atrial thrombi or tearing the fragile dilated chamber. Destruction of the valve under direct vision using a cardioscope was less promising. Associated observations on the operated dogs with relevance to patients included the radiological changes in the cardiac silhouettes that developed with different valvular lesions, the healing of pericardial and myocardial wounds, and the response of the heart to trauma.

With his increasing expertise and confidence in operating upon the canine heart, Cutler was ready when the first clinical opportunity rose. With the enthusiastic support of Viennese cardiologist Professor Karl Wenckebeck, then visiting the Brigham, a 12-year-old girl was accepted for surgery. She had a history of many colds and sore throats as a young child, but denied episodes of chorea or rheumatic fever. Her shortness of breath had progressively worsened during the previous

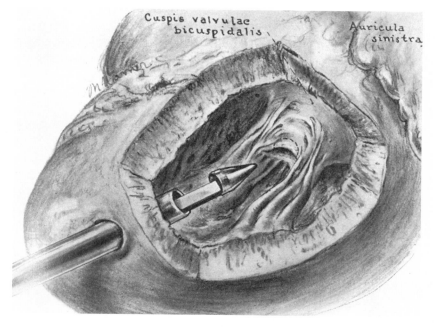

FIGURE 8.2   The valvulotome that Cutler and his colleagues developed to remove portions of calcific mitral valves via the transventricular approach (*J Expt Med* 1924, 40:375).

four years to the point where she could not lie flat comfortably. On examination she was slightly cyanotic. Her heart rate was rapid. The precordial region bulged, a thrill was felt and a loud diastolic murmur heard. On May 20, 1923, Cutler opened her tight mitral valve, the first such operation in history. He later described what occurred.

"At 8:45 a.m. the operation was commenced. A medial incision was made over the sternum from opposite the first interspace to within two inches of the umbilicus. Fingers of the right hand were then passed beneath the sternum and pericardium and pleura dissected away from it. The sternum was then split in the midline up to a point opposite the second intercostal space. Using slow and general retraction, the thorax was then opened outward, the pleura being swept back from the chest wall as it opened outwards by wet gauze dissection. The two halves of the sternum were held open by a rib spreader and a perfect exposure of the pericardium obtained. The pericardium was then split up its anterior surface almost to the very base of the heart, taking care to avoid the pleurae, which nearly met in this area. Next, the posterior pericardium and diaphragm were divided, permitting the bottom of the wound to open widely and expose the entire heart to view and manipulation.

"The pulse, which was 180 during the early stages of anesthesia, had dropped to 120, and the pressure had dropped from 110/50 [mmHg] to a systolic of 50. At times it was difficult to get any blood pressure reading whatever, and during such times the pulse was practically imperceptible. Realizing the heart muscle will stand severe trauma better if gradually initiated to its task, the heart was several times rolled out of its position with the left hand, allowing us to see more perfectly the left ventricle which is almost completely hidden by the dilated right ventricle and huge auricles. At this point about 1/2cc of 1:1000 adrenaline solution was allowed to drip over the heart, followed by some hot salt solution. At once the heart responded by vigorous and full contractions. This moment was seized as our more propitious one, and rolling the heart out and to the right by the left hand, the valvulotome, an instrument somewhat similar to a tenotome or a slightly curved tonsil knife, and the one with which we are most familiar in our experimental work, was taken in the right hand and plunged into the left ventricle at a point of about one inch from the apex and away from the branches of the descending coronary artery, where two mattress sutures had already been placed. The knife was pushed upwards about two and a half inches, until it encountered what

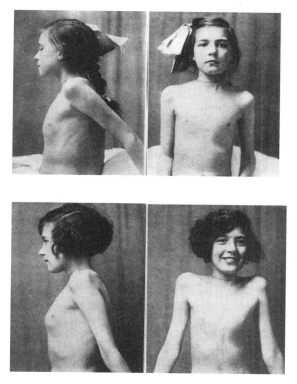

Figure 8.3   Cutler's patient before and after her successful mitral valvuloplasty (*Boston Med and Surg J* 1923, 188:1023).

seemed to us must be the mitral orifice. It was then turned mesially, and a cut made in what we thought was the aortic leaflet, the resistance encountered being very considerable. The knife was quickly turned and the cut made in the opposite side of the opening. The knife was then withdrawn and the mattress sutures already in place were tied over the point at which the knife had been inserted. There was absolutely no bleeding. Hot saline was dripped on to the heart, whose action continued good. The operation was over by 10:00 a.m."[9]

The patient improved considerably and she returned to a normal life before dying suddenly from recurrent stenosis four and a half years later. Emboldened by this success, Cutler performed similar procedures on three additional individuals. They died of "non-cardiac causes" 10 hours, 20 hours and six days later, respectively.[10] With this

143

experience, he, his co-workers, and a few additional pioneers, could claim that surgical intervention (12 instances in total by 1929) was warranted in particular instances of mitral stenosis and that further opportunities for cure should be exploited.

DURING THE NEXT SEVERAL YEARS, Cutler, Beck, and other investigators became increasingly conversant with the anatomy of the thorax of both dog and human and facile with operative approaches of the lungs, heart, and great vessels. He described at length the various transthoracic techniques he used to expose the heart, noted methods for handling and dislocating the beating organ, and identified means of repair of cardiac wounds. He characterized ventricular massage during a state of "suspended animation," and expended much effort in the experimental production of lung abscesses as part of an overall study of postoperative pulmonary complications. Following the lead of Edward Churchill at the MGH, his "favorite operation" became pericardiectomy after disease or trauma, a subject that he and Beck had examined extensively in laboratory animals.[11] While crediting a suggestion put forward years earlier, he was the first to propose formally (1927) that a

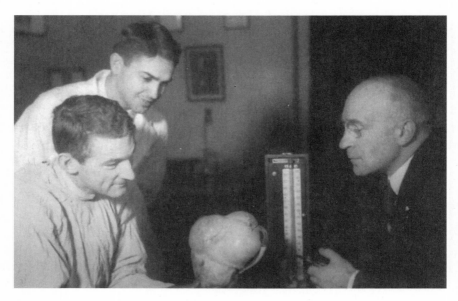

FIGURE 8.4   Cutler, a resident, and Burt Wolbach, professor of pathology.

patent ductus arteriosus could be ligated in children without other congenital anomalies.[12] One of his trainees, Robert Gross, successfully carried out the procedure 12 years later.

In an era when surgeons and physicians were just beginning to
believe that the diseased heart might be amenable to intervention or
repair, Cutler began to focus on the operative relief of angina pectoris,
a subject not even mentioned in the surgical textbooks of the time.
While appreciating the connection between chest pain and sclerotic
coronary arteries but unable to attack the arteries directly, Cutler's
interest in indirect approaches to treatment stimulated him to investigate two indirect approaches.

The first was cervical sympathectomy. Proposed in 1889 as a
means to relieve angina, the evolving rationale for the procedure was
complex.[13] Nervous impulses from the ischemic heart travel to the
adjacent sympathetic chain via small cardiac nerves. They are then conducted to the spinal cord through the first thoracic ganglion where
they evoke chest and arm pain. Theoretically, the heart could be isolated from its sympathetic supply by removing this and nearby ganglia
and dividing associated major nerves. Several surgical groups supported this idea by performing such operations in individuals with
angina.

Although Cutler reported enthusiastically in 1926 that the procedure prevented cardiac-associated chest pain in a series of his patients,
he became increasingly concerned that the effect of nerve ablation
could not be measured accurately in physiological terms. As in comparable situations in clinical medicine where pain is the primary symptom, precise analysis of specific symptoms must be studied directly, as
assessment in animals is impossible. About the same time, the Harvard
physiologist, Walter B. Cannon, showed that cats with a denervated
heart could survive without difficulty but that complete neurologic isolation of the organ could not be achieved without cutting the roots of
the upper *nine* dorsal nerves in addition to the sympathetic chain.[14]
This important observation eventually served to dampen surgical ardor
toward the concept of cervical sympathectomy, as removal of all affer-
ent pathways was, in effect, impossible.

An alternative strategy then came into vogue. With knowledge
accruing during the 1930s about the function of the endocrine glands,
reports were arising that hyperthyroidism could masquerade as heart
disease and produce anginal symptoms. In collaboration with Brigham

cardiologists Samuel Levine and Eugene Eppinger, Cutler reasoned that subtotal or total thyroidectomy would relieve the diseased heart of an extra functional load, particularly if the basal metabolic rate was already elevated.[15] Relief of symptoms would result. They initiated an extensive series of clinical studies to measure physiological changes after gland removal.[16] Elated by the early results of the operation, they even postulated that a hormone produced by the thyroid could act directly on the heart.

Cutler and Philip Shambaugh, a Cabot Fellow, embarked upon a series of experiments in dogs to define the relationship between the thyroid and cardiac function and to study the influence of complete gland removal on angina pectoris.[17] They passed a ligature beneath the left descending coronary artery and led it out the pericardium and chest wall via a glass tube. Traction on the end obstructed the coronary vessel of the awake subject, a situation manifested by stiffening of the forelegs and quickening of respiration. After determining that the response of the animal to coronary insufficiency was similar regardless of the presence of the thyroid, they modified their methods by passing the ligatures through pulleys and hanging small weights on their ends. Constant tension could thus be achieved without producing pain. Removal of the thyroid or the concomitant administration of atropine could block any discomfort that the dog showed following intravenous administration of adrenalin. The results of the studies supported the influence of adrenalin in promoting angina and suggested that the potentially beneficial effect of total thyroidectomy might be due to interference with a thyro-adrenal mechanism.

As neither the experimental data nor the clinical findings convinced Cutler as to the efficacy of the procedure, he encouraged his research group to pursue other ideas. One strategy included attempts to bring a new blood supply to the canine muscle. During studies on the production of pericarditis, Beck had conceptualized that newly formed vessels in the adhesions developing between the inflamed pericardium and the heart could provide an accessory circulation that could revitalize a poorly nourished myocardium. He also showed that muscle grafts from the ribs or pedicles of omentum brought through the diaphragm would adhere to the cardiac surface and create a small vascular supply.[18] He and others later adapted these experiments to patients. Following his research fellowship with Cutler, Beck completed his clinical training in Cleveland. Spending his entire career studying the heart, he became the first professor of cardiac surgery in the United States in 1952. A productive innovator and leader, his work in cardiac resuscitation and in revascularization of the heart was critical to this emerging field.

Another of Cutler's laboratory fellows, Mercier Fateux, performed a series of experiments designed to combine some of the ongoing concepts. When he cut selectively the small nerve branches that entered the heart directly to stimulate the coronary arteries but not the major trunks, ("pericoronary neurectomy"), 40% of the dogs died. He also found that occlusion of the descending branch of the left coronary artery inevitably caused death of the subject. But if he ligated the companion vein simultaneously to force open pre-existing collateral channels and increase arterial blood supply to the heart muscle, 40% of the animals lived.[19] With both pericoronary neurectomy and coronary venous ligation, the incidence increased to 87%. Fateux eventually reported the use of this approach in 16 patients, with relief of symptoms in the majority.

In reviewing the subject of treatment of angina pectoris in light of his own results and those of others, however, Cutler worried whether many of the putatively "improved" individuals actually had the condition to begin with. He decried the lack of complete follow-up data in most reports and, as noted, emphasized that the important psychic element associated with this disorder made it difficult to clarify accurately the end results of surgical palliation.[20] Increasingly, he felt it unfortunate that surgeons should explore any field in which they were not experts in diagnosis, mentioning specifically autopsy reports of persons with classical anginal symptoms whose coronary arteries were uninvolved by arteriosclerosis. His misgivings provide an interesting comment about a pattern that recurs intermittently throughout medicine as a whole: that enthusiastic and involved clinical investigators may widely herald therapeutic claims without fully supportive clinical or experimental data or adequate long-term assessment.

Although based upon trends prevailing at the time, the concepts of operative relief of angina by autonomic nerve ablation or thyroid removal were ill conceived. In retrospect, the effect of these procedures on a compromised coronary circulation was negligible. External revascularization of the myocardium with vascular pedicles from the chest wall as Beck had described, in contrast, persisted into the 1970s and is occasionally still used in patients with severe coronary disease as an adjunct to more direct measures. Not until coronary artery bypass grafting became routine a decade later, however, did Cutler's dream of effective surgery for angina pectoris more fully fulfill its promise.

CHAPTER 9

FRANCIS MOORE,
THE NEW CHIEF

BRIGADIER GENERAL CUTLER returned to the Brigham from Europe at the close of 1945, well aware that his advancing prostate cancer was responsible for his increasing fatigue and weight loss. Despite worsening bone pain that made movement difficult, he concentrated on meeting the protean challenges of his department. The academic careers of the young men who had just returned from the military, on hold during the years of conflict, required attention and support. Their needs had to be balanced with the demands of those who had remained at home and were more visible on the academic ladder. Some of the staff returned to their prior responsibilities, others moved to positions in other centers. It was a difficult and dynamic time.

Cutler husbanded many of his remaining energies as chief consultant in surgery in the Veterans Administration. This was a critical assignment, as the VA had experienced a gradual loss of interest by public and government alike between the two wars and a progressive decline in the academic credentials of its leaders. With the conclusion of World War II, however, a massive influx of veterans, often with complex medical and surgical problems, claimed attention. The solution advanced by the professor and his colleagues was to establish a close relationship between existing and proposed VA hospitals and university-associated teaching hospitals with their academic faculties and trainees. Repaying the debt of national gratitude to the veterans through conscientious medical care benefited all.[1]

His final months were replete with honors. The Secretary of War came to his house to award him the Oak Leaf Cluster. Despite requiring frequent blood transfusions, he gave his final lecture, *The Education of the Surgeon*, as President of the American Surgical Association and received the prestigious Bigelow Medal from the Boston Surgical Society for his broad investigative work.[2] His death at age 59 left a substantial void in international surgery.

FRANCIS DANIELS MOORE assumed his new duties as chief in 1948, a year after Cutler's death, replacing Quinby who had headed the department in the interim. Moore was already highly regarded both for his clinical knowledge and scientific contributions. One of the surgical interns at the time recalls his first sight of the new appointee at Grand Rounds. "I was seated high in the amphitheater and saw it all. Every dignitary [on the staff] had come and was seated. A couple of minutes before the appointed hour, a young guy, breathing a bit fast, came in the side door, turned to go up the steps to a rear seat, and seeing none empty, came down the stair and slid into the only remaining seat in the front row, between David Cheever and John Homans. Homans quickly turned to him and in his lisping voice said, loudly enough for most to hear, "Young fellow, you'll have to go up to the back. This theat ith retherved for the new profethor," to which the young man replied, 'I *am* the new professor!' "[3] A long-time Brigham physician later described the feelings of the faculty following his arrival. "After Elliott Cutler's demise, one would have thought that the surgical service might have a less visible, less flamboyant, less energetic chief. Not at all!"[4]

He grew up in comfortable surroundings near Chicago. Coming East to Harvard College, he made up for what he later described as a "less than spectacular" academic career by his increasing expertise in writing prose and in composing and playing music. As president of the *Harvard Lampoon* in his junior year, he and his friends became famous for purloining the Sacred Codfish from the State House in Boston as a prank. In a sequel, the following year they removed the Yale bulldog from New Haven to Cambridge, an event covered by the newspapers in detail for a full 10 days. Indeed, Handsome Dan II appeared on the cover of the March 1934 issue of the *Lampoon*, appropriately licking the foot of the statue of John Harvard. Moore's musical talents burgeoned at the Hasty Pudding Club, for which he and a colleague, Alastair Cooke, wrote a highly acclaimed show entitled *"Hades! The Ladies!"* After a successful local run, they took the production on a prolonged road trip around the country. Their adventures included tea in the East Room of the White House with Eleanor and Franklin Roosevelt, the latter once a member of the Pudding chorus.

He entered Harvard Medical School in 1935, one of a limited number of applicants who could afford the $400 tuition during the depression years. "When at mid-year I had done fairly well, the Dean of Admissions told me, 'Moore, you surprised us. You belonged to a lot of those college drinking clubs and I didn't think you would amount to a damn.' With this sobering thought to support me, I was able to face the subsequent years, my self-confidence intact."[5] Of the 110 members of the medical school class, 18 later became professors of surgery, apparently stimulated and guided by the renowned surgical faculty of the time. Moore, too, entered the field he was later to describe as "organized optimism."

Substantive changes in education and professional development occur slowly. Indeed, Moore's residency training at the MGH appeared little different from that which Cushing had experienced nearly four decades before. For the first few months of internship, for instance, the primary task of the new "pups" was to collect and analyze, early in the morning, the urine and feces of selected patients, as directed by their more experienced seniors. "Our equipment for this simple but important (albeit odiferous and inelegant) task was primitive in the extreme and left an unmistakable mark on the décor of our tiny attic laboratory in the Bullfinch Building. Urinalysis consists in part of the spinning down of urine in the centrifuge and examining the sediment under a microscope for signs of infection. This required a small centrifuge, with little pointed tubes that were apt to break at the tip if dropped too heavily into the centrifuge. If a tube filled with urine had a tiny hole in it and was twirled at a rapid speed, the walls of the room and everything at a certain height around the wall would be decorated with a narrow brown strip, this being the even distribution of urine around the room at the precise level of the spinning centrifuge. I wore an apron."[6]

The new interns walked circumspectly a few steps behind their seniors on daily rounds. Transfusions had only recently progressed from the direct donor-to-recipient method via paraffin-lined tubes to the collection of blood from family members in bottles. The addition of sodium citrate prevented clotting and allowed storage. The pups carried out the cross-matching and typing themselves. They picked the instruments for the next day's operation, assisted at surgery and performed increasingly complex and closely supervised procedures as they gained seniority over the next 3–5 years. They also administered anesthesia, initially (like Cushing) unsupervised. "It was shocking to me, and I still look back on it as a dereliction of the high standards of our surgical education that I was suddenly confronted late at night with an anesthesia machine, valves, cranks, and canisters of nitrous oxide and oxygen, and was expected to proceed, untutored, to induce anesthesia and put the patient 'to sleep.' At night, hurried, harried, and tired, with no help. That I and my fellows got through this without causing any deaths was pure luck. My own revolt against this practice as a pup was simply to state clearly that I would never give another night emergency anesthetic unless I (and the other interns to come) could give it safely under experienced supervision. By the look in my eye, that hospital administrator must have realized that he was dealing with a fairly determined pup."[7]

ON THE NIGHT OF November 28th, 1942, nearly 1,000 people packed the Coconut Grove, a popular nightclub near the Boston Common just off Charles Street. Suddenly, fire broke out. Toxic smoke billowed from curtains, furnishings, and artificial palm trees. Tables blocked most of the emergency exits. Once removed from the carnage, the victims were taken as quickly as possible to all the hospitals in the city. Moore was one of the two surgical residents on-call in the emergency room of the nearby MGH. The treatment rooms and hallways were suddenly filled with burned patients, many already dead. Of the 114 unfortunates who crowded together on all the available floor space, only 39 remained alive after the first few hours. Completely untrained for such a catastrophe, the staff quickly tried to separate those potentially salvageable from those who were obviously dying. While they could provide acute treatment with fluid resuscitation, transfusions, and local care, they could do little to relieve the almost ubiquitous respiratory distress.

Manifestations of the burns were revelations to those treating the patients, as many of the initial signs and symptoms that the patients displayed were unexpected, poorly understood, and often unresolvable.[8] A large number of individuals in the nightclub had suffocated as the fire rapidly consumed oxygen from the closed space. Others died of carbon monoxide poisoning within a few hours. Still others died of irritant gases produced by burning paints and plastics. To that point, the management of severe burns had changed little throughout the ages. Indeed, the subject was barely discussed in surgical texts of the time. Early treatment remained limited to topical application of a variety of substances to prevent fluid loss. Silver nitrate was used to seal the open areas, tannic acid to promote scab formation, gentian violet for its potentially bacteriostatic properties. Later, the inevitable infections developed. Penicillin was not obtainable initially and only in small amounts thereafter. Rehabilitation was formidable, as limited coverage of the burned surfaces with skin grafts took weeks or months. Those surviving often developed severe contractions from the intense scarring.

It was later determined that a total of 490 people died in this catastrophe; 440 survived. Indeed, burns comprising over 30% of the surface of the body were inevitably fatal. While an overwhelming and disheartening experience for the physicians involved, the tragedy opened a new area in patient care that continued to fascinate the young surgeon throughout the remainder of his career. Moore and his mentor, Oliver Cope, quickly initiated a series of important studies on the physiology of burns and the resultant alterations in the homeostasis of the body.[9] Their contributions and the accumulating body of work from investigators ongoing in many centers have improved patient care to such an extent that half those with 80% burns currently survive.

Moore finished his abbreviated residency in the months following Pearl Harbor. As chronic asthma kept him out of the military, he entered practice with Leland McKittrick, a busy surgeon at the MGH. His clinical interests quickly turned toward solving two common problems. Surgery of the overactive thyroid gland was a significant challenge facing many surgeons of the time. While Cutler had excised normal thyroids to reduce the pain of angina, and those in other groups and clinics had become highly experienced in removing large hypoactive goiters, operations on the edematous, inflamed, and highly vascularized hyperactive glands remained difficult and dangerous. As a result, the need to normalize thyroid function to prepare hyperthyroid patients for surgery was an important issue. The young surgeon quickly exploited the relatively novel idea of using thiourocil, the latest of a group of drugs developed since investigators two decades before had first recognized that dietary iodine could alter thyroid activity.[10] Additionally, radioactive iodine was just becoming available. Taken up avidly by the overactive tissue, the isotope killed functioning cells. This advance would make the operation unnecessary in many cases.

Peptic ulcer, Moore's second interest, also affected many individuals throughout society, a debilitating condition characterized by auto-digestion of local areas of the upper gastrointestinal tract by excess acid-pepsin from the stomach. While ulcers of the stomach were apparently more common in the nineteenth century, the incidence of duodenal ulcer increased as the twentieth century progressed. Relatively large numbers of patients developed complications of the condition. Unrelenting pain occurred most frequently, although free perforation of the duodenal wall, obstruction of the pylorus with scar tissue, or hemorrhage from the ulcer eroding into an adjacent artery were common. Indeed, during my residency in the late 1960s, 3 or 4 individuals with duodenal ulcer were admitted each week to the surgical service. We operated immediately upon those with perforations. If they were obstructed, we placed naso-gastric tubes on constant suction to empty the dilated stomach and allow the acute swelling to subside. As intravenous nutrition had not yet been described, many lost dangerous amounts of weight. If bleeding was significant, my fellow house officers and I would spend often futile nights pulling out huge clots of blood via a naso-gastric tube, then instilling iced saline into the stomach in an effort to stop the bleeding. Most went on to surgery.

As obstruction remained particularly poorly controlled by medical means, occasionally surgeons in the 1890s began to bypass the swollen and scarred duodenum by suturing a loop of small bowel to the most dependant portion of the stomach. This arrangement not only appeared to correct the problem but was considered a physiological improvement, as alkaline bile from the intestine would enter the stomach directly and neutralize the acid. The procedure, gastroenterostomy, was relatively successful in older patients whose acid production was low. In younger patients, however, gastric acid flooding directly onto the small bowel segment not infrequently produced an unexpected problem, "the marginal ulcer." Hemorrhage often resulted. And even more sinister, the ulcer often burrowed into the adjacent colon, forming a fistula that connected all three structures. This "complication of ulcer surgery in the period 1890–1930 carried a truly impressive mortality for its repair."[11]

More extensive operations came into vogue in subsequent decades, increasingly centered around removal of portions of the stomach and reconnecting it to the small bowel to restore the continuity of the gastrointestinal tract. The surgery was not always easy. Even Zollinger, a master technician, commented on one of his less-than-calming experiences as chief resident. "[My] second rotation on [Cutler's] service gave me the opportunity to perform more advanced surgery. For example, he made it possible for me to perform a gastric resection for intractable duodenal ulcer. I was to follow his teaching that a limited antrectomy [removal of the distal portion of the stomach] followed by anastomosis to the duodenum was in the best interest of the patient. After the antrum was resected, I was left with a duodenum about 4 cm wide and a stomach at least two times that width. Although I had assisted Dr Cutler perform this procedure a number of times, I was temporarily panicked about how I could bring these two structures of such unequal size together with safety. I sent word to Dr Cutler that I needed suggestions as to how to proceed. He sent back the message, 'Young man, never take anything apart that you can't put back together again!' We did get it together and the patient survived."[12] Many of us have been in the same position!

It occurred to Moore early in 1943 that division of both vagus nerves plus a minimal gastric drainage procedure might be a practical alternative to gastric resection in patients with peptic ulcers. Several nineteenth-century experimentalists had shown that their division not only decreased the secretion of acid in gastric pouches in dogs but that the animals remained healthy thereafter. In the 1920s a few European surgeons reported the results of cutting the nerves in patients with peptic ulcer disease. They also noted that as one of the additional functions of the intact vagi is to open the pyloric sphincter. As surgical interruption of the nerves cause it to close, adjunctive gastric drainage was necessary. Considering these older findings, Moore targeted an appropriate patient for operation. Before he could carry it out, however, Lester Dragstedt, a surgeon and gastrointestinal physiologist from the University of Chicago, reported the results of vagotomy in several individuals.[13] The benefits were as predicted.

Despite this scoop, this subject remained a long-term interest for the young surgeon who, with several of his colleagues, continued to make important early contributions to the field.[14] Indeed, over the next 15 years stimulation or inhibition of acid-producing cells by antral hormones was proven to be dependant on the pH of the stomach. With this increasing understanding, he and a growing number of other surgeons began to carry out the less extensive and morbid vagotomy and pyloroplasty procedure, cutting the nerves then dividing the pyloric muscle to ensure gastric emptying. This operation ultimately became the approach of choice for intractable peptic ulcer, although many of my teachers and their peers throughout the country still favored the more extensive gastric resections for some years thereafter. Cutting individual nerve branches to the stomach, selective then highly selective vagotomy, gradually replaced truncal vagotomy in many series. For years the surgical literature was replete with discussions and arguments about new and refined operative treatments of the condition.

But regardless of all the time and effort, surgery for peptic ulcer became progressively less frequent. Not only did the incidence of the disease decline in the population at large but the introduction of potent pharmaceutical agents in the 1970s to inhibit production of hydrochloric acid effectively reduced many of the symptoms and many of the complications. More recently, a bacterium, *Helicobacter pylori*, has been identified as responsible for many cases, an observation that won its discoverers the Nobel Prize in 2005. Surgical intervention of this once almost endemic condition has been replaced by treatment with pills.

MOORE HAD MIXED EMOTIONS about his future career as he completed his training. With a background both in surgery and in basic science, and with the opportunity either to pursue private practice with McKittrick or to continue his investigations into the physiology of burns and of the stomach, he realized he was "part surgical practitioner, part surgical scientist, never wishing to abandon completely the joy of surgery despite the pull of the laboratory."[15]

A born teacher, his leadership abilities also became quickly apparent. As chief resident he had emphasized impeccable professional conduct and intellectual honesty to his juniors as well as the compelling need for operative skill and conscientious patient care. While technically expert, he "converted himself to a teaching surgeon who could help juniors and let them feel unconstrained but subtly keeping safety and control: a higher skill."[16] Already in the forefront of several areas of surgical care and perhaps sensitized by his unexpected "race" with Dragstedt, he stressed that priority of discovery was unimportant. "No scientific laboratory works alone. There has been an unfortunate emphasis on the concept of priority in research. Competitive instincts seek to establish that the individual achievement has been the 'first.' A moment's reflection will tell us this is not important. It is much more important to see clearly the importance of some new development and

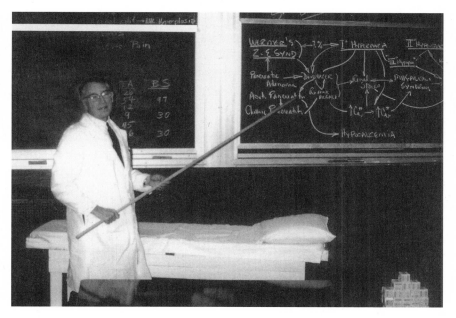

FIGURE 9.1   Francis Moore, the new professor, in 1950.

carry out study or education which helps exploit a new field to its fullest."[17] With his obvious personal and professional attributes, the Brigham Trustees picked him as Cutler's successor. He was 34 years old.

The incumbent soon discovered that much needed to be accomplished in his new institution, as he later noted when characterizing its differences with the MGH. "The MGH was large and strong at that time, while the Brigham was small and much weakened by the war and an aging senior staff. It had only 250 beds, compared with the 850 beds at the MGH and the surgical department was taking some hard hits. Not only had Elliott Cutler died, but other prominent surgeons there, notably David Cheever and John Homans, were close to or at retirement age. Nobody was doing cardiac or thoracic surgery, and there was no one in charge of several of the other surgical specialties (gynecology, ophthalmology) at the Brigham. Some specialties (neurosurgery, orthopedics) were shared with nearby hospitals. Bob Zollinger had left to take over the service at Ohio State.

"On the other hand, the Brigham could hold its head up pretty well. While much smaller than the MGH, it had been responsible for many advances, ranging from the introduction (under Harvey Cushing) of an entirely new field, neurological surgery, to the publication of a new, richly illustrated how-to book, the *Atlas of General Surgical Operations* by Cutler and Zollinger. This bestseller was used extensively (surreptitiously even by the residents of the MGH) and avidly read by other surgical residents throughout the world. The Brigham was a haven of learning for students and residents. And in 1948 it had a young, brilliant, newly appointed Chief of the Department of Medicine, George W. Thorn. The possibility of working as Thorn's opposite number was very attractive."[18] In addition, a productive relationship with the head of pathology, Gustaf Dammin, was to prove of immense benefit to all.

The practical realities, however, were unnerving. The financial position of the hospital was tenuous. The income from the Peter Bent Brigham trust was nearing its end. As many of the patients were indigent and could not pay, there was talk of bankruptcy or even of merger with the MGH. The fortunes of the department were diminished by years of war, the prolonged absence of a chief, and a paucity of young and productive staff members. But even during the brief tenure that remained to him before his death, Cutler had wisely incorporated several individuals of manifold talents into the faculty. In place when Moore arrived were Robert Zollinger and Engelbert Dunphy in general surgery, Hartwell Harrison in urology, and Richard Warren and Chilton Crane, who were beginning their forays into vascular surgery. David Hume was becoming interested in endocrinology and in the novelties of kidney transplantation. Joseph Murray, already promised a position by Cutler, was about to enter the residency program in preparation for further training in plastic surgery. Carl Walter was continuing his work on surgical asepsis and blood bank technology. Robert Gross and Charles Hufnagel were actively investigating the correction of cardiac abnormalities and the replacement of vascular segments in the Surgical Research Laboratory.

Specialization in surgery was poorly developed at the Brigham despite gradually spreading throughout many institutions after the war. Moore's philosophy on this topic differed somewhat from the more generalist concepts of his predecessor; indeed, years before he had seen Cutler "perform (in a single day) an operation for a brain tumor, a hys-

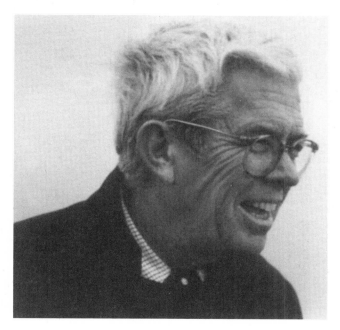

Figure 9.2   John Brooks.

terectomy, and a colon resection for cancer." It had also become clear from care of the wounded that only physicians and surgeons expert in a given body area or organ system could advance treatment of specific disease states. "Everyone is against specialization except the patient. The patient always seeks the most expert care."[19] As a result, he had to make several appointments quickly to broaden the scope and capabilities of his faculty.

He brought John Brooks with him from the MGH to be chief resident. Brooks would become a lifetime colleague, supporter and confidant. Having attended Harvard College and Harvard Medical School, he took a residency in surgery at Roosevelt Hospital in New York City after his wartime service. He then joined Moore as a research fellow to study the effect of vagotomy on duodenal ulcer, later publishing extensively on this subject. He was a "tall and physically strong man, and his usual good cheer was often punctuated with a marvelous reverberating laugh. His opinions were generally not hard to make out as they often came to the fore early in a conversation and then were not easily changed. Although, in the course of a busy and demanding day, he may have appeared gruff to some, his underlying disposition was sunny, and he enjoyed life and good fellowship immensely."[20] Active as a general surgeon at the Brigham throughout his career, he devoted much time and effort to teaching, advising, and mentoring the residents.

Brooks was responsible for many practical aspects of running the department. As head of the residency program, he organized and assigned coverage of the various surgical services with a firm but light touch. This role was especially problematic during the years of the Vietnam War when so many residents were entering the draft and replacements were arriving from other surgical programs. I recall clearly such an instance. I had been scheduled to begin a less-than-arduous rotation in the emergency room upon return from the one-week vacation allotted to us each year. Within moments of my entering the hospital, however, Brooks informed me that he had scheduled me to rotate a second time to Dr. Harken's exceedingly demanding and stressful cardiac service. Any considerations I had entertained for a relatively normal life, however transient, were dashed. With a twinkle in his eye and knowing full well my feelings, he patted me on the shoulder and wished me well! There was no debate.

The new subject of organ transplantation sweeping the Brigham in the 1950s and 1960s influenced his clinical interests toward the grafting of thyroid and parathyroid tissue. His expertise in gastrointestinal diseases, particularly of the pancreas, encouraged him also to consider the increasingly apparent problem of diabetes. While the life span of diabetics had been markedly prolonged since the introduction of insulin, they were beginning to develop unexpected and devastating long-term complications. Indeed, the routine use of the hormone transformed the disease from an acute and sometimes lethal condition to a chronic one, with many patients developing blindness, vascular insufficiency, neuropathy and renal failure. As a result, increasing numbers of investigators began to consider reversing these sequelae by transplanting functioning pancreatic fragments or even insulin-producing islets of Langerhans.

While occasionally scientists had attempted such steps decades before, Brooks revitalized the concept by performing a series of pancreatic autografts then allografts in dogs, and finally by transplanting pancreatic grafts of stillborn infants to their diabetic mothers. He was one of the early investigators to use millipore chambers in the circulation to protect the islets placed within from destruction by the host responses.[21] His studies of the possibilities of pancreas transplantation for diabetes culminated in a 1962 monograph on the subject, *Endocrine Tissue Transplantation*. Unfortunately, neither the times nor the methods then available were ready for such departures although other investigators, particularly at the University of Minnesota, persisted and gradually opened this field.

Brooks had broad interests. Highly visible in surgical circles, his wisdom, good sense, and gentle humor endeared him to his colleagues and to generations of house staff. He served his university in many ways, including his long tenure as surgical chief of the University Health Services. It was always interesting for us residents to care for some of the Harvard faculty transferred by him from Cambridge to the Brigham for surgery; their hospital experience, we were often amused to note, did much to deflate their sometimes vast academic egos. In fact, his three decades at the health service, caring for everyone from students to professors, provoked one of the faculty to quip: "He who's not been cut by Brooks, lacks essential Harvard looks!"

For years he cruised the Maine coast in a series of blue sloops called *Callina*. At the end of the season he often invited residents to sail the boat from Bar Harbor to her winter berth in Manchester, Massachusetts. This was always an adventure. We flew in a small commuter plane to Maine to meet him at the boat yard. It was invariably cold. We would then sail throughout the night on 4-hour watches. A dedicated New Englander, all he would serve to eat was peanut butter sandwiches—not even hot tea against the unrelenting chill. Character building, he would tell us, with the twinkle in his eye. During his memorial service years later, Robert Osteen, a member of the surgical staff, reminded us that Brooks, ever the dietary Puritan, had even resisted broadening the array of food served at the annual Brigham cocktail party at the American College of Surgeons meeting from its traditional cheese and cracker format!

Moore recruited one of his own teachers from the MGH to strengthen the emerging specialty of gynecology in his new department. A highly effective leader with broad surgical expertise, Somers Sturgis advanced substantially the developing field of endocrinology as it related to female hormones, sterility, fertility, and cancer of the ovaries and uterus. He perfected endometrial biopsy to determine the precise stage of the menstrual cycle in women about to undergo operations or hormone treatment. He was the first to transplant the ovary. One of his major contributions was to open the generally unspoken subject of a woman's emotional involvement in her reproductive function, writing eloquently about the psychological aspects of surgical removal of the uterus and ovaries and the resultant endocrine changes. A gentle, soft-spoken, and caring figure, a talented sculptor and artist, he was an important innovator in the emerging field of gynecology.[22] Indeed, many of us gained considerable operative experience in carrying out such procedures on a multitude of patients. Gynecology became a separate department in 1970.

ANESTHESIA ALSO REQUIRED urgent attention. Since Boothby had left the department in 1916, nurse anesthetists had administered the majority of anesthetics. In 1947 Quinby appointed William Derek to head the new division; he remained for five years then departed after three weeks notice, taking many of the nurses with him.[23] As a result, Moore suddenly found himself crossing and criss-crossing the country in search of a substitute. The hunt became virtually a full-time job, particularly as the specialty was underdeveloped in the United States in the post-war years and many anesthesiologists were unwilling to relinquish private practice to enter salaried positions in teaching hospitals. Fortunately, a few relatively well-trained academic physicians were beginning to enter the field and contribute to the increasingly relevant subjects of respiratory physiology, pharmacology, and associated biosciences. Leroy Vandam was one of these. Located at the University of Pennsylvania, Moore convinced him to join the surgical faculty at the Brigham. It was a fortuitous appointment.

Vandam was an ex-surgeon who had entered anesthesia after losing an eye. Very much his own man, he stood up to sometimes aggressive surgeons without qualm. His high personal standards caused him, at times, to react ferociously against what he considered inadequate or slipshod efforts by his residents or staff. One noted: "It took me some time to realize, when I met his gaze under such circumstances, that the eye with the kindly expression was the glass one!" Breathing a new spirit into the subject, he stressed that not only should the modern anesthesiologist choose, administer, and monitor suitable drugs and fluids during operation, he should be a compulsive clinical observer,

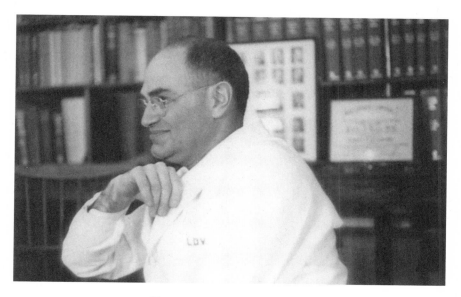

FIGURE 9.3   Leroy Vandam.

record pertinent information, resuscitate and treat respiratory changes, and be a teacher and investigator at the same time.[24] Surrounding himself with talented colleagues, he separated his group from surgery in the 1970s to form its own department. This schism evoked many pointed conversations between Vandam and Moore, two powerful and outspoken individuals. Despite it all, however, they remained lifelong friends and supporters.

"Dr. Vandam was an inspiration and a role model for everyone who trained or worked with him. He was not only an anesthesiologist, but a complete and consummate physician. His highest priority was to attest to the human condition and to alleviate suffering, anxiety and fear, the omnipresent concombinance of physical illness, and to blend his ministrations with the best that science and technology had to offer. His credo was simple and direct: he strove for perfection in every detail and demanded excellence not only from his staff, but primarily from himself. Patients and their families felt safe in his hands, knowing that he understood their vulnerability and that he would do everything humanly possible to assure a good outcome."[25] As a member of many national committees, he helped to shape and define the role of anesthesia in the late twentieth century.

In addition to his own significant clinical contributions and scientific investigations, he influenced the field substantially throughout his teachings and as a demanding editor-in-chief of the journal, *Anesthesiology*. A knowledgeable historian about the development of his subject, he had also trained as an illustrator, supplementing his excellent text, *Introduction to Anesthesia*, with his line drawings. Taking up water color painting later in life, his works became recognized nationally and were featured frequently on the covers of the *Journal of the American Medical Association*. During the summers he took anesthesia call at the cottage hospital on Nantucket. We residents once heard the startling news that the Brigham telephone operators had kept Vandam waiting too long on the line one Sunday afternoon when he wanted to speak with someone about a burned patient. Finally connected to the hospital administrator, he delivered a terse and furious opinion of the matter then promptly transferred the patient to the rival MGH. Heads rolled on Monday!

My own experience as a patient anesthetized by Vandam remains vivid in my memory. A young attending surgeon, I was playing squash with a colleague late one afternoon. At that time, no one wore protective glasses. In reaching around me to return a shot, my opponent struck my eye with his racquet. While I still had some vision, we both realized that the injury was severe. In the Brigham emergency room, the ophthalmologists confirmed that the eye was ruptured and that part of the iris was protruding from the defect. Operation was necessary. Dr. Vandam soon arrived to administer anesthesia as it was his rule to officiate at all surgical procedures performed on staff members. Several medical students were in tow. Telling me that he was going to "intubate me awake," he administered curare. And indeed I was awake, paralyzed, and able to hear him explain the proceedings as he showed my vocal cords to the students. Unable to communicate or to breath, I could only hope for the best. For years, he continued to maintain that the approach was the safest. I shudder at that experience to this day.

ALTHOUGH NEUROSURGERY THRIVED at the Children's Hospital under Franc Ingraham, the lack of attention to adult care was all too obvious to Moore on his arrival. The new professor asked one of his medical school classmates to fill the gap. Donald Matson was recognized as a scholar before his graduation, having already published several papers. Inspired by Ingraham to enter the specialty, he soon became responsible for neurosurgical care in the European Theater of Operations under Cutler's overall leadership. Completing his residency after the war, he began to treat complex neurological cases at both the Brigham and the Children's Hospital. A consummate physician, "he had a way of approaching the patient, the patient's problem, the operation, the patient's family, the pathology, the biochemistry and the sociology, joining them all together effectively, with gentleness, humanity, lack of false pride, willingness to consult others, and in one of the most difficult fields of surgery, with remarkable effectiveness."[26]

In addition to his clinical load, Matson spent much time examining the secretion, absorption, and metabolism of the cerebrospinal fluid, a subject of investigation introduced decades before by Cushing and Weed. Matson's interest came from his observations on the gradual loss of higher integrative function in children with hydrocephalus, a condition in which the fluid produced continuously in the brain cannot drain into the spinal canal because of anatomical or functional abnormalities. Intracranial fluid builds up. Although not the first to devise a conduit around a localized point of obstruction, he is credited with techniques to relieve communicating hydrocephalus by removing a kidney and draining the excess fluid from around the brain via a plastic tube that emptied into a ureter retained after sacrifice of one of the kidneys.[27]

Moore described the operation. "The very first patient (1948) that had an operation of this type was a little girl of eight, who, following a severe head injury, had developed a communicating type of hydrocephalous due to obliteration of the subarachnoid space. A rather large plastic tube conduit was placed between the lumbar subarachnoid space and the ureter, the kidney being removed. The child got along very well. Pressure was relieved. Waning mental function returned. Within a few weeks it was possible to close the defect in the child's skull, a repair in which Dr. Matson was also experienced from his treatment of wartime head wounds. He published this as a case report, noting the obvious limitation that it was but a single case, yet with course and recovery sufficiently remarkable to justify publication."[28] This success introduced a novel and innovative method of treatment for such children.

Possessing far-ranging talents, Matson became a leading neurosurgical figure. Within a few years, he published his experience on 100 subarachnoid-ureteral shunts, and then his results of another 100 patients who received ventriculo-ureteral shunts.[29] Recognized internationally as the Matson Procedure, variations of the techniques are used to this day. His early use of plastic that could be retained indefinitely in the body opened the way for further surgical applications including artificial heart valves, arterial prostheses, and the replacement of hips and other joints with synthetic devices. He also worked with colleagues at MIT to develop an effective valve for his shunt. With George Thorn, he was one of the first to use replacement adrenal steroids in hypophysectomized patients. His pioneering forays into a variety of neurosurgical problems, sometimes to the consternation of his residents, substantially advanced the field.

A serendipitous but critical offshoot of the Matson procedure was the sudden availability of a normal kidney from the hydrocephalic children. In the early days of renal transplantation at the Brigham, Murray and Harrison grafted these kidneys into immunosuppressed recipients, an important impetus to a novel program that would evolve into a worldwide venture. Unused organs were brought to the laboratory of John Enders at Children's Hospital who was developing methods to grow poliovirus on primate tissues. Culture of human kidney cells enhanced the development of a vaccine against that dreaded affliction of childhood.

Matson died at the height of his powers from a progressive neurological disease, possibly a slow virus contracted from one of his patients. The authors of a memorial essay noted well his place as a clinical investigator, laying out at the same time his views of the role of the surgeon-scientist: "In human biology, the pathway from the laboratory to the bedside passes the milestones of the three 'D's: Discovery, Development, Delivery. Basic science is Discovery, be it insulin, poliovirus, DNA, protein structure and synthesis, or molecular immunology. Delivery is the repetitive application of procedures to many patients. Between Discovery and Delivery there is an important middle ground. Dr. Matson's work was located there, in Development. It is work designed to bring to practical usefulness some new facts or concepts developed by the physical and biological sciences. In that sense, developmental work is engineering.

"Innovative application of the new concepts and techniques to the care of the sick have recently been epitomized in surgery by the development of tissue transplantation, open heart operations, shunts for hydrocephalus, vascular grafts, aortic aneurysm repair, total hip reconstruction, cranio-facial remodeling, middle ear rebuilding, and re-attachment of the retina. Each has marked a new era of hope in human illness and relief of suffering for many. These are all examples of developmental biology or engineering. This has been true of all the development of surgery since the time of Lister: the intelligent development of methods, born in laboratory science, to the care of the sick.[30]

THIS IMAGINATIVE AND PRODUCTIVE staff, part inherited from Cutler, part gathered by Moore, eased itself into place with the change in leadership of the department of surgery. Moore later summarized the philosophy that he brought to his faculty. It remains remarkably relevant in the present era of managed care. "At a time when society is questioning the relevance of the highly specialized teaching hospital, using elaborate equipment and a large, specialized staff for acute care, and is looking towards some sort of community goal, it is well to remember that at the center of the teaching hospital there are people who actually treat and cure major diseases that cannot be treated or even approached anywhere else in the world. Their patients come from any community. Those that treat them are individuals who know how to use strong academic institutions, major hospital resources and an expert staff."[31]

CHAPTER 10

INVESTIGATORS ALREADY IN PLACE

Despite the changing departmental dynamics, several imaginative investigators continued to pursue their studies in the Surgical Research Laboratory during Cutler's final years and the period after Moore's arrival. The contributions of three individuals in particular became significant in the history of modern surgery. Robert Gross involved himself for nearly a decade in designing operative techniques to correct congenital heart defects in children, and with Charles Hufnagel, developed methods to preserve and store arterial allografts to bridge vascular defects too large to be brought together primarily. Hufnagel was the first to treat aortic insufficiency in patients using a novel intra-arterial ball valve device. David Hume examined both the hypothalamic control of the pituitary and the endocrine changes that occur with stress. Their contributions sustained the Brigham research enterprise at a high level in a difficult time during and after the war and provided a substantial background for operative advances and applied biologies that Moore and his faculty were to carry out over the next decades.

Gross entered the field of surgery in a somewhat circuitous fashion. Robert Bartlett, a Brigham resident later working with him at Children's Hospital, describes the progression of events. "When Robert Gross was a chemistry student at a small college in Minnesota, he read [Cushing's] Pulitzer Prize winning book, *The Life of Sir William Osler*. [He] was fascinated and read the book over and over again. He became obsessed with the idea of becoming a doctor, becoming a surgeon, and studying with Cushing in Boston. He applied to Harvard Medical School and was accepted. At the first opportunity he

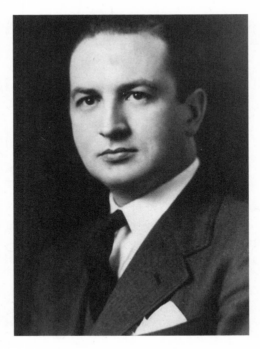

FIGURE 10.1   Robert Gross.

crossed Shattuck Street to the Brigham to the operating suite, to the
gallery in Room 2 to watch the famous Cushing operate. Midway
through the first operation Cushing looked up and said 'Who are you?'
'I'm Robert Gross, a freshman medical student. Ever since I read your
book . . .' 'This is no place for medical students, go away,' said Cushing. Gross was dismayed but worked hard at his studies and applied to
Cushing for surgical residency 4 years later. [Although] Cushing
refused him, he entered the pathology residency at the Brigham. Three
years later when Cushing retired, [the chief of pathology] convinced
the new chief Elliott Cutler to put Gross into the surgical residency,
and he excelled in the position."[1]

During his years of training both in surgery and pathology, Gross
developed an enduring interest in the disorders of infants and children, eventually joining the surgical staff of both the Brigham and the
Children's Hospital. The early relationship between these institutions
had not been close. From the time Children's had opened its doors, the
institution had dedicated its clinical and research activities toward

pediatric care and training. While some of its house staff already had credentials in adult care, little interaction with the Brigham occurred. This situation began to change in the 1920s, however, with the construction of an overhead bridge across Shattuck Street to connect the two buildings. Within a few years and encouraged by Franc Ingraham, the surgical chiefs, Cutler and William Ladd, formed a joint training program in which selected house officers took a pediatric surgical internship followed by two years of general adult surgery before completing their requirements at Children's. Cutler later described this increasingly productive liason.

"I should like to report at this time that we are making progress in the contemplated union of the surgical internships of the Children's Hospital and the Peter Bent Brigham Hospital. We now lack, for the benefit of our house staff, training in the recognition and care of many of the embryological defects seen in children, for which surgery is a benefit; and at the same time, interns now obtaining their surgery largely at the Children's Hospital need some experience in the care of the common diseases of the adult which cannot be studied in a hospital restricting itself to the preadolescent period. A joint internship of possibly two and a half years duration should provide a more adequate training for the young surgeon than is commonly available and it is our hope that this can be worked out before the next intern examinations fall due."[2]

Gross took full advantage of this dual arrangement. During his time in pathology, he had examined a number of infants and children who had died with congenital anomalies and had become increasingly convinced that corrective surgery could not infrequently be possible. Cardiovascular abnormalities, particularly of the great vessels entering and leaving the heart, intrigued him specifically. The patent ductus arteriosus was one of these.

The young surgeon began to define the anatomy of the great vessels near the hearts of laboratory animals, their relationship to the recurrent laryngeal nerves that supplied the vocal cords, and the possibilities of surgical manipulation. Having worked out a precise operative approach to the ductus in 20 dogs, he, with the support of cardiologist John Hubbard, operated on the first patient on August 26, 1938. Gross was chief resident. "A girl of seven and a half years had a known patency of the ductus arteriosus and beginning cardiac hypertrophy. In the hope of preventing subsequent bacterial endarteritis and with [the] immediate purpose of reducing the work of the heart caused by the shunt between the aorta and the pulmonary artery, the patent ductus was surgically explored and ligated. The child stood the operative procedure exceedingly well. The most objective finding, which indicated that the serious loss of blood from the aorta into the pulmonary artery had been arrested by operation, was a comparison of the pre and postoperative levels of diastolic blood pressure. Prior to operation the daily blood pressure showed an average diastolic level of 38 mmHg as compared to a postoperative diastolic level of 80 mmHg. This was the first patient in whom a patent ductus arteriosus has been successfully ligated."[3] She went home in seven days.

Gross nearly lost his position at Children's by performing the operation. Bartlett tells the story in more detail. "When chief resident at the Children's Hospital he proposed to the chief, William Ladd, to try an operation to close a patent ductus. Ladd said 'Absolutely not. First of all there is no way to operate on the chest of children. Secondly everyone knows that operating around the heart or great vessels is always fatal.' Ladd forbid him to even consider the operation. Gross waited until Ladd went out of town—to Europe by boat—and brought in two children on which to operate; two in case one died. He performed the operation with the nurse anesthetist giving positive pressure mask anesthesia. He ligated the ductus, and the bounding pulmonary artery quieted down, and the child recovered successfully. When Ladd returned from Europe, he was furious that Gross had performed the operation against his instructions. He fired him, the chief resident. Others in the Children's Hospital implored him to bring Gross back. They could see the successful outcome and knew all too well the usual outcome. Finally Ladd relented and invited him back to complete the residency. In typical fashion, Gross responded, 'No, you fired me and I'm building a barn. I'll return when the roof is on.' "[4]

This single case changed dramatically long-held opinions about the potential of surgery of the heart and great vessels, previously limited to occasional repair of stab wounds, relief of restrictive pericarditis, and Cutler's few forays into opening stenotic mitral valves. Indeed, the success of Gross's procedure injected reality into the long-standing debate about correction of the condition and stimulated the formation of surgical laboratories around North America to pursue related investigations. A Boston surgeon, John Monroe, had introduced the concept that a patent ductus could be treated in a lecture in 1907 to members of the Philadelphia Academy of Surgery. Operative intervention was considered in occasional patients for years thereafter but was never carried out despite improvements in surgical technique, relatively effective anesthesia, and the introduction of intratracheal intubation to control respirations during operative entrance into the chest. In 1936, a published report described 92 autopsies of patients with the condition.[5] None had other congenital anomalies. Finally, on March 6, 1937, John Strieder, a surgeon at Boston University across the city, closed the patent ductus of a young girl with sutures. Although her symptoms disappeared, she died four days later of acute gastric dilatation.[6] Gross had not known of Strieder's attempt.

Following his first success, he performed his operation in a series of patients. All patients did well until the fourteenth, a girl who thrived initially but collapsed two weeks later during a party at her house. The ligature had cut through the fragile vessel, producing massive hemorrhage. Indeed, Gross's concern about such a possibility had caused him to test a variety of materials to close the ductus, including thick silk or cotton tape, and wrapping the occluded portion with cellophane to increase regional scarring. He never again ligated a ductus but devised a clamp that did not crush or cut the thin wall of the dilated conduit. Following its division, he closed the vascular cuff meticulously with a continuous silk suture, reporting the successful use of the method in a further group of patients.[7] From these beginnings, Gross's operation has saved the lives of many children over the world.

Despite a general lack of interest and expertise in vascular repair by most surgeons, a handful of investigators like Gross began to broaden their researches during the 1940s to include the correction of a variety of congenital defects in children that involved the heart and great vessels. Treatment of another important developmental anomaly, coarctation of the aorta, was particularly challenging, as the constricted segment had to be removed and the vessel reconstituted. In coarctation, the aortic segment is narrowed at or near the origin of the ductus. The affected portion is usually localized but may occasionally involve a longer arterial segment. Although some patients may live a normal life with this condition, its complications may be fatal in others even as adults. In addition to aneurysm, rupture and infection, hypertension of the upper part of the body may produce cerebral hemorrhage and cardiac failure.

First by himself and then in collaboration with a surgical resident, Charles Hufnagel, Gross redesigned his vascular clamps to obstruct the

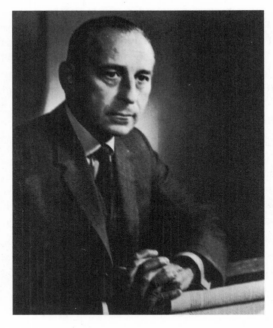

FIGURE 10.2   Charles Hufnagel.

thoracic aorta of anesthetized dogs by shortening the blades of straight intestinal clamps then fitting the ends with a small interlocking peg to keep them in position when closed. Longitudinal splits and cross marks were cut in the jaws to prevent slippage. The jaws were then sprung to grasp and occlude but not injure the vessel wall. With the aorta obstructed above and below the coarctation, the investigators could divide the vessel and reconstruct it with interrupted sutures of fine oiled silk on small needles. While they initially abutted the three arterial layers directly to each other, intima to intima, media to media, adventitia to adventitia, they did not include the intima in their suture, as they considered it undesirable to leave silk within the vascular lumen. They quickly abandoned this method, however, because of bleeding upon removal of the clamps. They next everted all layers of the vessel ends with a continuous suture. Although an improvement, unexpected hemorrhage still occasionally occurred.

A third method of vascular repair, described the year before by Alfred Blalock at Vanderbilt, was to employ a continuous mattress suture to evert the entire thickness of the aortic wall. Bleeding was negligible and no constriction at the site of repair occurred. Using Blalock's approach, Gross published the results of the experiments several years later. "These experiments have been less extensive than originally planned, and have been curtailed by the exigencies of the war. Nevertheless, they have progressed to a point where we believe that a method has been devised for the treatment of coarctation of the aorta in human subjects."[8] And in an addendum to the paper, he mentioned his first two patients. He had carried out his first clinical repair on June 26, 1945, using mattress sutures.[9] The child died shortly following removal of the clamps, possibly because of a sudden release of metabolites into the circulation from the anoxic tissues. On his second attempt the following week, however, he removed the clamps slowly. This child and subsequent children did well.

He was not aware that a previous visitor to his laboratory who had seen him create and repair an aortic coarctation in dogs was working on the same problem. Clarence Crafoord, a professor of thoracic surgery in Stockholm, was a highly experienced surgical investigator and the first to suture the ductus shut instead of ligating it. He had also shown that animals could withstand finite periods of ischemia of their peripheral organs if blood flow to the brain was maintained. Finding that he could safely cross-clamp the aorta of patients for as long as 30 minutes, he performed his first repair of an aortic coarctation on October 19, 1944 and his second 12 days later.[10] Crafoord and Gross published the descriptions of their cases about the same time.

Gross always kept more than one project in his vision. He was the first to treat another congenital heart defect, aorto-pulmonary fistula, then described and repaired various vascular rings that constricted the esophagus or the trachea. In the days before cardiopulmonary bypass, he devised a well technique to allow closure of intra-atrial septal defects. But effective methods to bridge the long arterial defect that remained after removal of an extensive coarctation, still escaped him. Older investigators had used tubes of glass, gold or paraffin-lined silver as vascular substitutes. In the laboratory Hufnagel was designing and placing a permanent, rigid prosthesis into the thoracic aorta of dogs. At the same time, others were examining the use of venous segments from the animal itself (autografts), or from members of the same (allografts) or different species (xenografts) to replace arterial defects, using Vitallium cuffs for the anastomosis. Unfortunately, while feasible in experimental models, segments of peripheral vein of suitable size did not exist for the adult human patient, while the metal cuffs and rigid prostheses constricted the growing aortas of children.

Aware that others had transplanted fresh pieces of aorta between dogs years previously, Gross and Hufnagel began to investigate means to preserve vascular segments for later use as grafts. Beginning with the culture of canine arteries in test tubes, they examined the effectiveness of quick freezing allografts and occasional xenografts in appropriate media, then maintaining them at temperatures just above freezing.[11] They removed appropriate vessels from the donor animals 1–6 hours after death and cold-stored them as long as 42 days before use. Emboldened by their experimental results, Gross implanted segments of human arterial allografts frozen in nutrient broth into a large series of patients with coarctions too extensive to join primarily after resection.[12]

New methodology emerging in the 1950s broadened the experience. Hufnagel preserved pieces of aorta in helium before freeze-drying. Gross x-radiated frozen arterial grafts, a direct outgrowth of studies carried out nearby at the Massachusetts Institute of Technology on the effects of high energy rays on biological materials.[13] Preservation of the vessels in formalin met with less success. In 1951, Felix Eastcott, a Brigham research fellow who would later assist on the first carotid endarterectomy in a human and become professor of surgery at St. Mary's Hospital, London, evaluated with Hufnagel the significance of the rate of freezing on the arterial wall.[14] They concluded that a two-phase method using direct immersion in liquid nitrogen for rapid freezing followed by prolonged deep freezing gave the most satisfactory results.

Within a few years, the arterial allograft was generally considered to be the most satisfactory replacement for arterial defects. Thrombosis occurred infrequently and an adequate supply of vascular segments of various sizes could be obtained postmortem. One ex-resident, John Rowbotham, described their use in the Korean War. "I had the best Army job possible as chief surgeon in a MASH behind the front lines. We did lots of artery grafts on extremities which we deemed salvageable. Our 'bank' was a Mason jar kept in the fridge [that contained] saline laced with penicillin. We took our donor grafts from cadavers who had died of head wounds and who had 'clean' abdomens and legs. We had segments of artery anywhere from one to four inches long, and would pick the one we needed with forceps when the head nurse

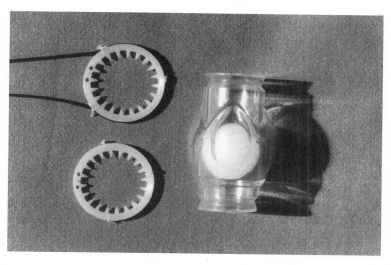

Figure 10.3   The first ball valve to be implanted in a human with aortic insufficiency, showing the multifixation rings for the aorta.

unscrewed the cap and held the jar over our table. Crude, but it worked."[15] However, as long-term follow-up data gradually accrued, it became apparent that the incidence of late stenosis or aneurysm formation rose to unacceptable levels. Increasingly, surgeons interested in the problem directed their investigative energies toward the development of prosthetic grafts, primarily to replace abdominal aortic aneurysms in adults.[16] Vinyon-N cloth, then orlon, nylon, Teflon and Dacron appeared and were tested. The latter materials have become standard in modern vascular operations.

Gross remained a major figure in the developing field of pediatric surgery. In addition to his substantative contributions to the operative correction of congenital abnormalities of the heart and the great vessels, he described innovative approaches to a broad spectrum of surgical diseases of children. His books on the subject written during a busy clinical and investigative career, *Abdominal Surgery of Infants and Childhood* (1941, with William Ladd), *Surgery of Infancy and Childhood* (1953), and *An Atlas of Children's Surgery* (1970), are classics.

In addition to his extensive collaborations with Gross on the development of vascular grafts, Hufnagel became expert in the origins and pathophysiology of aortic insufficiency, designing a variety of ball valves housed in a rigid prosthesis to correct the condition. He placed the devices in the thoracic aortas of dogs, anchoring them in place with multi-fixation external rings in lieu of sutures, a technique still used in cardiac surgery.[17] Carrying out a series of trials to determine the optimal materials, he initially tested methylmethacrylate for the housing and plexiglass for the ball, then devised a silicone rubber ball molded over a hollow nylon center of critical weight to allow its activation by small changes in blood pressure. He implanted his first prosthesis in a patient with aortic insufficiency in 1952, eventually placing them in over 20 afflicted individuals.[18] I remember seeing one of these individuals when I was a resident. The seating noise of the valve was audible to those of us standing at the end of her bed. Indeed, when we placed our hands on the metal bed frame, the transmitted vibrations were obvious. While very distressing and leading to some suicides, the difficulty was solved in later designs. Some patients with hitherto fatal aortic insufficiency lived for long periods. Hufnagel's unique contributions to the repair of valvular heart disease led the way toward an entirely new area of treatment. He also stirred the beginnings of a new field by using his developing vascular expertise to transplant kidneys in dogs with David Hume, one of the surgical residents.

He left the Brigham to become chief of surgery at Georgetown University in 1950, possibly in part because he felt that Gross was using his ideas too freely. He took his experimental animals with him. Moore later described the eventful transfer of the dogs with "clicking valves" from the Surgical Research Laboratory to Washington, DC. "To study these devices (a ball valve that could be used within the heart) he [Hufnagel] placed them in the aorta in a large series of dogs in our laboratories at the Harvard Medical School. When he accepted a job as professor at Georgetown, he asked me if he could [keep] the dogs. Of course I agreed, because these dogs were extremely valuable, priceless. There were no others like them anywhere in the world. Also they had become pets of the laboratory team. Their long-term follow-up over the course of years would be necessary to determine the extent of wear and tear on the ball valve. So he loaded all his dogs into a small trailer to drive them from Boston to Washington. When he reached northeastern Connecticut, he needed to make a pit stop at a filling station. As Hufnagel disappeared into the restroom, the attendant heard a dog barking in the trailer, and thought an animal probably wanted out to irrigate a local tree. So, thinking there might be one or two dogs inside, he opened the trailer door. About 25 dogs bounded out, barking and sniffing and wagging their tails delightedly. This part of Connecticut about halfway between New York and Boston is largely uninhabited, quite a wild place for this canine diaspora. Yapping with joy at their release from the noisy trailer, the dogs disappeared into the hills.

"This would have been a terrible loss to science and cardiology had it not been for the ingenuity of Hufnagel, the dismay of the filling station attendant, and the willingness of the local dog catchers to cooperate in an unusual medical adventure. All the dog officers were given stethoscopes and were instructed to hold down any dog they caught, stray or otherwise, and listen to his chest. One of the dogs had returned to the trailer, and the dog catchers were all given a chance to listen to what a ball valve sounded like, clicking back and forth in the chest with every heart beat. Unmistakable. If the dog clicked, keep it. It wasn't long (about a week) before all the dogs were rounded up and sent on their way to Hufnagel's laboratory in Georgetown University. This

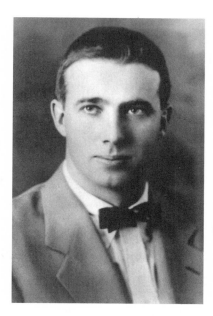

Figure 10.4   David Hume.

179

work, these valves, and a study of these dogs in the inventing of a new device had given him a secure place in surgical history."[19] Hufnagel continued his innovations at Georgetown, designing effective leaflet and disk types of cardiac valves.

David Hume joined the Brigham as a surgical intern in 1943; a note from his internship folder noted that he "talks fast but makes good sense."[20] He joined the staff in 1947 following his residency, a few months before Moore's arrival as chief. The new professor recalled his first abbreviated conversation with his young faculty member: (Moore) "What is it that you are working on and what do you need?" (Hume) "The pituitary and money." (Moore) "Fine, so lets go get it." Knowledgeable, hard driving, argumentative, and iconoclastic, Hume immediately began work. His interest in the "master gland" was timely, as it complemented George Thorn's ongoing investigations into the function of the adrenocortical hormones. In fact, Hume's researches continued an enduring theme at the Brigham that had begun with Cushing's own involvement with the pituitary and would relate well to the new biology that was to emerge from Moore's laboratories.

By 1900, the endocrine glands had been identified as a unique component in the homeostasis of the body. Controlled by secretions from specific areas in the brain, these structures release hormones directly into the circulation that affect the behavior of different tissues. Cushing had discovered that the pituitary was responsible for an unexpected variety of functions by relating unusual physical traits and physiological disturbances in his patients to over-secretion or under-secretion of particular cells within its substance. It was evident that the structure produced factors that could stimulate the adrenals, the ovary, the testes, or the thyroid, as well as having a profound effect on body growth, particularly of bone. If abnormalities occurred, giantism or dwarfism could result. In addition, its central location in the brain immediately below the optic nerves could, if it became enlarged, produce local visual disorders unrelated to the central mechanisms of vision. By 1908, shortly after Roentgen's discovery of x-ray, lateral films of the skull of afflicted individuals could be taken to detect enlargement or erosion of the surrounding bone. With this new diagnostic technique, abnormalities could be detected, a half-century before accurate chemical methods became available to assess levels of hormones in the blood. Following the publication of his book on the pituitary, Cushing and his co-workers in Boston continued their investigations into the physiology of the gland. Indeed, the first paper they published from the Surgical Research Laboratory involved its role in carbohydrate metabolism.[21] Hume's investigations into the regulation of the pituitary by the hypothalamus, a higher structure in the mid-brain, took this knowledge further.

He had graduated from Harvard College six years after Cushing left the Brigham for Yale. And like the professor, his college career was not brilliant. Although the two men never knew each other, Cushing and Hume had several features in common: a capacity for hard work, a creative imagination, personalities at times difficult, the institution of new fields of surgery (Cushing, neurosurgery and Hume, transplant surgery), and an enduring interest in the pituitary gland. Failing to be admitted to Harvard Medical School, he attended the University of Chicago where he became particularly impressed with the studies of Dr. Charles Huggins, a surgeon who was beginning to relate the influence of the endocrine system to tumor growth or regression. Huggins later (1966) received the Nobel Prize for his work on the hormonal treatment of prostate cancer.

Hume entered his internship, stimulated by Huggins's observations that "certain nerve cells in the lower portion of the mid-brain looked as though they might not only be nerve cells but secretory cells, like endocrine glands."[22] He hypothesized that this area of the brain, the hypothalamus, might influence the function of the pituitary and, ultimately, the endocrine system itself. He studied this subject for the next decade, initially by stimulating specific portions of the brain remotely via a small radio transmitter that gave off electronic impulses to receivers placed in the neck of dogs. With this device he could activate electrodes located in particular central sites. Despite no evidence of pain or other sensation by the awake subjects upon transmission, widespread changes in endocrine function occurred with stimulation of the hypothalamus. Unfortunately, he had to curtail these experiments, as his transmissions interfered with radio-contact between the control tower at Boston's Logan Airport and Eastern Airline pilots trying to land their planes.

He next attempted to isolate some factor from portions of the brains of animals that could activate the pituitary itself, eventually showing that adrenal hormones could, in turn, stimulate the pituitary in a "feed-back" manner.[23] Related studies involved assessment of adrenocortical function in surgical shock in dogs and in patients with severe burns, and the relationship between the adrenal glands and protein loss following fractures in rats. He went on to develop an assay for ACTH in the blood, of special interest to Thorn for use in his patients with adrenal tumors, pituitary disease and other endocrine disorders.

William Ganong, a physician also working in the surgical laboratory, continued to enlarge and refine the ongoing studies during Hume's subsequent absence in Naval service. In addition to other results, Ganong showed that gradual bulk reduction of the pituitary affected endocrine function differentially. Adrenocortical function disappeared last, long after thyroid and gonadal activity was undetectable.[24] This finding suggested that only a small amount of retained pituitary tissue was necessary to stimulate the response of the animal to injury, a reaction intrinsic to its survival. His experiments were also critical for Thorn who had described a means to analyze changes in pituitary function with stress and for Moore in his developing studies of the systemic effects of surgical trauma.

Hume's investigations occurred during a period in which Moore was examining body composition and the response to injury, "during the decade when understanding of the endocrine-metabolic response to surgery was undergoing a rapid phase of development. His [Hume's] work evolved throughout this expanding phase as one of the important connecting links in the growing chain of knowledge. When an individual is injured, impulses pass through nerve cells to the brain and from thence communicate themselves to the endocrine glands. This modification in endocrine activity maintains the normalcy or 'homeostasis' of the individual. In terms of clinical surgery, these studies have dealt with the connecting links between the wound and the man as a whole."[25] Within a few years Hume became head of the department of surgery at Virginia Commonwealth University. As one of the early pioneers of the new subject of kidney transplantation, his contributions and those of his faculty were far ranging. His untimely death in 1973 left an important void in international surgery and surgical research.

THE WORK OF THESE THREE investigators and others in the department, combined with Moore's early studies on body composition and the effects of injury, provided a solid groundwork for the productivity and innovation in a variety of the biosciences that would be sustained over the following decades.

CHAPTER 11

CONCEPTS, STRATEGIES, AND ADVANCES

MOORE FACED A VARIETY of new dynamics permeating the practice of surgery during the early years of his tenure, many stemming from lessons learned in wartime. The operative challenges of World War I, often carried out in suboptimal conditions, had primarily involved limb amputations and relatively limited repair of abdominal and cranial injuries. Individuals who survived were removed to non-combatant areas for long-term recuperation. Surgeons in World War II stabilized the acute injuries of soldiers in the mobile field hospitals that Cutler and Zollinger had instituted, then evacuated them as expeditiously as possible for further surgical intervention or rehabilitation. Intravenous fluid transiently restored circulating volume; the newly available pure human albumin, much from Harvard laboratories, saved lives. Antibiotics were appearing. Increasingly conversant with such innovations, surgeons returning to civilian life became bolder in their approaches to a variety of disease states and conditions. More radical surgery for cancer, the beginnings of effective vascular reconstruction, and operations on the heart were among the results.

Surgical research, one of the new professor's major interests, was also experiencing a renaissance. Interested practitioners traditionally had carried out their scientific investigations on a part-time basis funded by private sources. With a few exceptions, the contributions of surgeons to biological knowledge had been relatively few and generally technical in nature. The exigencies of war, however, altered substantially the direction of surgical thinking toward more sophisticated and directly applicable areas of study. Clinical conundrums demanding solutions included treatment of hemorrhage and shock, the care of burns, and complex reconstruction of patients who had survived severe

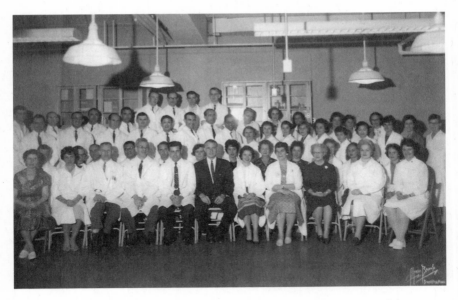

FIGURE 11.1   The laboratory crew in 1960. Joan Vorhees, supervisor of the
Surgical Research Laboratory, Margaret Ball, guiding light in Moore's Brigham
laboratory, and Doris Lewis, Moore's long-time secretary, sit to his left.

deforming injuries. The need to understand the acute alterations in
fluid and electrolytes developing after injury and the later use of body
components in healing grew in importance. Moore spent much of his
career investigating these metabolic changes and defining means to
normalize them.

One of his first priorities was to acquire an appropriate laboratory
to continue the studies of body composition he had begun three years
before at the MGH. As the space needed to be organized around
patients, its location needed to be in the hospital and separate from the
animal facilities. Fortuitously, a large area near his office became available. An intervening library/conference room became the center for
research meetings for the planning and discussion of the torrent of
investigations that soon began to pour forth from his expanding
research group. In addition to John Brooks, he had brought Margaret
Ball with him from the MGH to direct his laboratory. A graduate of
Radcliffe College and a chemist from Oliver Cope's laboratory at the
MGH, she quickly became a driving force behind the ongoing projects,
ruling, organizing, and educating generations of research fellows.

Caryl Magnus, a statistician responsible for the analytical work and for the preparation of the radioisotopes, soon joined her. There was little concern about the risks related to the handling of the radioactive material; the extra product was often poured down the drain.

Moore quickly announced the direction that his efforts would take. "Surgical research comprises three areas of endeavor. One, the technical field, covers 'how to do it.' The second, the clinical field, covers the question 'what are the statistical results?' The third field is essentially an area of biological science and deals with the question 'what is the individual patient's reaction to surgery and his disease?' In the first of these areas, the Surgical Service here has always been active and effective. The long and brilliant record of the Laboratory for Surgical Research and the publication of Dr. Cutler's *Atlas of Surgical Operations* bespeak the effectiveness of this institution as a vehicle for technical research and education. Although the number of surgical cases operated upon at the Brigham Hospital rarely approximates the statistical series published from larger hospitals and group clinics, the papers published annually from this service on the clinical results of various surgical approaches bear witness to our activity in the second area of follow-up studies. Study of the biological response of the patient to trauma, disease and surgery is a relatively new and rapidly expanding field of endeavor. Neither the Laboratory for Surgical Research nor the wards alone can provide the setting for this type of work. It is research which requires on the one hand a carefully run and closely supervised clinical service and on the other hand laboratory quarters where chemical analyses or isotope studies may be run with ease, accuracy and abundance. It does not require large numbers of patients; it is a form of investigative activity 'made to order' for the Brigham. At the time of this writing, the new surgical laboratories have not been finished but the busy program of construction is a welcome harbinger of the imminent realization of our hopes in this area. This laboratory, when completed, will be a unit in which a wide variety of research problems may be carried out, and indeed we look for increasing collaboration between this laboratory, the Laboratory for Surgical Research, and the hospital wards themselves."[1] Indeed, the proximity of these areas to each other was a significant factor in Moore's continuing productivity throughout his tenure.

Adequate support is always an issue for investigators who must go to considerable efforts to finance their laboratory enterprise. Cushing had maintained his research efforts through sparse departmental money sometimes supplemented from his own pocket. While the medical school had appropriated some funds for Cutler's investigative activities, these were "entirely inadequate to defray the heavy expense of the type of work carried out there."[2] Private donors helped, particularly Harold S. Vanderbilt, who had given a large gift in 1924 to underwrite the experiments in cardiac surgery by Cutler, Beck and Levine.

Little monetary relief for the ongoing investigations was forthcoming during Cutler's absence during the war, although Quinby, the acting chief, had held on. Moore described the rather tenuous situation. "One of Dr. Quinby's outstanding problems dealt with the financing of the Laboratory for Surgical Research. The increasing cost of even the simplest items and the increasing grade of research activity in the laboratory and the medical school had mounted in the past three years to the point where the usual budgetary sources could not possibly swing the load. Without knowledge of the person or plans of the new surgeon-in-chief, it was impossible for Dr. Quinby to make the type of commitment essential in obtaining research grants from government, industry or private foundations. Faced with such a situation, many would have sought the easy solution of cutting down the activities of the laboratory, closing off some of the projects, battening down the hatches, and weathering out the storm until the new chief arrived. Such a course did not appeal to Dr. Quinby and instead a sizable sum of money was transferred from other sources to the laboratory and with this transfusion the laboratory continued its healthy course of activity. The busy productive program funded there was a delight to the new incumbent; our gratitude is herewith recorded."[3] The contributions of Gross, Hufnagel, and Hume were ample compensation.

As scientific research is inevitably expensive, Moore had a pressing need for start-up funds. When he arrived at the Brigham in 1948, for instance, he discovered to his consternation that the dogs used in the laboratory had cost $17,074.74 for the year. It might be mentioned in this context, however, that the bill for rats and their board for my own laboratory experiments in 2001 was as much as $10,000/*month*. But despite the emptiness of the departmental coffers, several sources of support were gathering. The new professor enthusiastically acknowledged the "unrestricted funds" given by generous donors who included Vanderbilt, the Boston financier F. L. Higginson, and other local philanthropists. Inscribing his first book, *The Metabolic Response to Injury*, to Higginson, Moore wrote appreciatively: "I know this all seems very abstruse and obtuse—yet I want you to have a copy and I want again to tell you of our abiding gratitude for your generous help." Pharmaceutical companies expressed interest, although the professor made it clear to their representatives that the funds must be unrestricted and that direction of the research by industry was unacceptable. Most importantly, federal bodies including the military services, the Atomic Energy Commission, and the Public Health Service were becoming intrigued with his studies with radioisotopes and on the effects of injury on the metabolism of the body.

The Coconut Grove fire had focused sharply Moore's interest in the events occurring within the body after physical insult. To define these changes, he began to consider the biophysics, quantification and applicability of the radioisotopes that had become available since the development of the cyclotron in 1937. As a medical student he had been impressed with the work of the MGH physician-scientist Fuller Albright on metabolic changes related to endocrine dysfunction. Receiving a small stipend from the National Research Council, he joined the laboratory of one of Albright's colleagues, Joseph Aub at the Huntington Hospital, a small cancer hospital near the Brigham. An expert in nutrition, Aub was also a pioneer in the use of isotopes in research. Moore and his laboratory colleagues soon defined a potential clinical role for the new materials by creating sterile abscesses in rabbits, then locating them with radioactive dyes. Cope and he then used these markers to examine alterations in capillary and lymphatic permeability of burned tissues in animals and in patients. The results led to an understanding of the hidden but substantial loss of fluid into injured and inflamed tissues.[4] The young investigator later acknowledged Cutler's interest in these studies. "In the early years of my research work when I was at the Huntington Hospital, Elliott Cutler was extremely enthusiastic and had me into his office to tell him all about it. He was thrilled to think that a young surgeon was learning how to use radioactive isotopes. I am sure that had he remained around and had remained active, he would have continued to be a good friend."[5]

Their wartime experiences had reinforced the impression of many thoughtful surgeons that some of their most urgent problems involved "dangerous inaccuracy, inadequacy, and often disastrous ineffectiveness of supportive care for patients who had sustained severe injuries, burns, or major operations."[6] It was clear that more accurate knowledge of water and salt distribution was needed to improve the situation, not only in normal individuals but following serious physiological perturbations. Under contract from the Navy for such studies, Moore's experiments at the Brigham focused increasingly upon the bodily changes following operative trauma and convalescence of surgical patients. "The rapidly widening horizon of medical research with radioactive and stable isotopes of the common biologically important elements has long since come to include the sphere of surgery."[7]

Research already ongoing in his new department may have stimulated pursuit of these subjects further. Hume was beginning to define the hypothalamic-pituitary pathway and the endocrine response to injury, Dunphy was examining experimental traumatic shock and replacement therapy, and Walter's prior successes with intravenous treatment was improving patient care dramatically. In the department of medicine, George Thorn's examination of the function and application of adrenal cortical hormones to various disease states richly complemented these efforts.

There was some precedence for Moore's investigations into the physiology of the surgical patient. German scientists at the end of the nineteenth century had considered the influence of fever as an integrated somatic reaction to a systemic stimulus. Cannon at Harvard had explained the generalized changes developing after injury by showing that stress may activate the adrenal medulla to produce large amounts of epinephrine and norepinephrine. This "flight or fight" response, in turn, triggered other metabolic perturbations. Between the world wars, an Edinburgh veterinarian, David Cuthbertson, noted that large fractures caused rats to lose significant protein as manifested by elevated levels of nitrogen excretion. The "alarm reaction" described by Canadian biochemist Hans Selye related psychosocial stresses with physiological changes via activity of the endocrine glands; hypertension, duodenal ulcer, and arthritis could result. Fuller Albright's analysis of protein loss in Cushing's Syndrome caused him to draw parallels with the observations of Selye and Cuthbertson on the reactions of the body after injury. As these separate threads of knowledge began to be drawn together into a comprehensive whole, the influence of the adrenal corticosteroids in the conversion of protein to carbohydrates appeared increasingly to be the common denominator.

No accurate means of estimating these dynamics existed. Patients died in shock from inadequate circulating volume or drowned from overzealous infusion of fluid. If the traumatic insult was large or infection developed, they lost substantial body cell mass. Moore postulated that quantification of the various somatic components would lead to understanding of the changes occurring during the spectrum of surgical illness. The principle of measuring selectively individual compartments of the body by the dilution of specific isotopes opened several pathways to investigate and calculate accurate fluid and salt requirements after injury. Determination of "total body water, extracellular water, blood volume, the total mass or weight of body cells, total sodium and total potassium" became possible.[8] Radioactive chromium, developed in Thorn's department, was used to assess red cell volume. Plasma volume was quantified with Evans blue dye.

In 1946, Moore first established the principle of "body composition" by calculating the dilution of known amounts of deuterium or tritium in the body to measure total body water. Alternatively, animals were killed, weighed, and desiccated to absolute dryness, then weighed again. The change in mass after removal of all water from the subject correlated exactly with the isotope dilution results. He and his group then measured total weight of sodium and potassium, checking and rechecking the data with various techniques. They calculated the values for humans in similar fashion by studying patients who had willed their bodies for such studies. The use of these methods spread quickly to other laboratories throughout the world where they were reexamined, modified, and improved. And almost three decades later, one of Moore's research fellows used the most current isotope technology to re-analyze the early results using a different animal model.[9] The correctness of the original data was confirmed.

He and his expanding research team continued to broaden the scope of their investigations. Studies of acid-base balance included description of the alkalosis that may develop after multiple blood transfusions and following injury. They defined the relationship between endocrine function and fluid and electrolyte changes developing after trauma, systematically examined the differential effects of surgical injuries of varying magnitude and their relationship to gender and age,

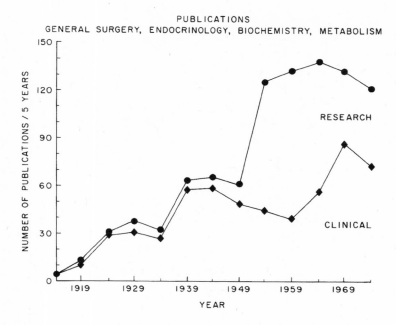

FIGURE 11.2   Number of publications on general surgical subjects from the
department during the tenure of the first three professors. The burst of productivity
under Moore is striking.

and scrutinized the re-assimilation of body proteins during healing and
convalescence.

The nutritional needs of surgical patients also became a sustained
interest. A hitherto normal individual undergoes a period of starvation
during the acute phase of injury. Survival is dependent upon mobiliza-
tion of protein from muscle and its transformation into carbohydrate-
based energy. As the sickest patients are often unable to eat, nutrition
administered parenterally must be adequate to replenish bodily tissues
during healing and convalescence. Initially reviewing the subject in
1948, Moore expended much effort over the next two decades in
determining the effectiveness of various infused intravenous substrates.
He was well aware of Albright's unsuccessful efforts to provide intravenous nutrition with protein hydrolysates and glucose in patients who
failed to thrive despite these supplements.[10] The large number of clinical and research publications produced by those working on these sub-

jects during Moore's tenure attest to the sustained productivity in the department.

Despite the significant contributions of the Brigham investigators to this emerging field, however, the most convincing data emerged in 1968 from the laboratory of Jonathan Rhoads and his colleagues at the University of Pennsylvania in highly controlled experiments in dogs.[11] They showed that total parenteral nutrition could support the normal growth of puppies, and even allow uneventful parturition in the adults. "Almost immediately after this publication, the word on total intravenous feeding spread over the world, finding a special usefulness in infants born with disorders of the gastrointestinal tract, in people suffering severe wounds, and in those debilitated because of cancer or chronic infection. Few events in the field of nutrition and metabolism have changed worldwide practice as much as this publication by Rhoads and his group."[12]

Douglas Wilmore, one of Rhoads's co-workers, later joined the surgical faculty at the Brigham to continue his nutritional studies. Over the following decades, he defined the role of specific factors in treating the critically ill and discovered, contrary to accepted dogma, that glutamine was a conditionally essential amino acid and that growth hormone was fundamental in alleviating the debilitating response to injury. When these substances were administered intravenously together or in combination with other nutrients, they could support the lifetime needs of patients with short bowel syndrome or other nutritional deficits. The influence of the experimental and clinical data generated by Rhoads, Moore, Wilmore, and colleagues in other centers opened a new direction in patient care that has been highly significant to the scope and safety of surgery.

Moore summarized his clinical data with descriptions of the research methods used in 1952 in a book, *The Metabolic Response to Injury*, authored with Margaret Ball. In 1959, he published a more detailed monograph, *Metabolic Care of the Surgical Patient*, in which he described 32 patients with a broad range of surgical conditions and discussed in detail their metabolic alterations during carefully defined stages of injury and healing. Within a few years, the group published further concepts and results in *The Body Cell Mass and its Supporting Environment*.

The professor later summarized the overall theme of his long-term investigations. "In that search for the unifying principles which underlie all scientific inquiry, the concept has become firmly rooted that following trauma [or injury], there occurs a characteristic and invariable disorder, marked in its progress by clearly recognized way stations, a fixed route from illness to recovery."[13]

He had already embellished these thoughts in the Introduction of *Metabolic Care of the Surgical Patient*. They say much about the man and the philosophy he preached constantly to his trainees. "The fundamental act of medical care is assumption of responsibility. Surgery has assumed responsibility for the care of the entire range of injuries and wounds, local infections, benign and malignant tumors, as well as a large fraction of those various pathologic processes and anomalies which are localized in the organs of the body. The study of surgery is the study of these diseases, the condition and details of their care. The practice of surgery is the assumption of complete responsibility for the welfare of the patient suffering from these diseases. The purpose of this book is to provide a guidebook for metabolic care in surgery. The focus is entirely on the care of the patient."[14] *Metabolic Care* became a huge

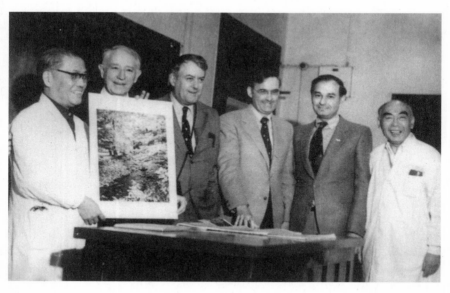

FIGURE 11.3   Moore and his group in Beijing in 1982, at the time he was presented with a Chinese translation of his text, *Metabolic Care of the Surgical Patient*. In return he is presenting our hosts with a picture of the Wyoming mountains. (left to right) Professor Tsen, Moore, Couch, Tilney, Hechtman, Wu.

commercial success, was translated into many languages, and was on the bookshelves of surgeons throughout the world. I well recall a visit to China with Moore years later, shortly after the end of the Cultural Revolution. At a small but formal ceremony in Beijing, our host presented him a copy of the book that had been translated, unbeknownst to him, into Chinese. The book changed many aspects of peri-operative care.

Many who worked in that laboratory have vivid memories of the experience. Murray Brennan, for instance, one of the many research fellows during Moore's tenure, arrived from New Zealand in 1969. He later joined the residency program and has ultimately become a highly regarded chairman of surgery at Memorial-Sloan Kettering Cancer Center in New York. He described the ongoing investigations. "For the 'lab rats' working in the bowels of the Brigham, it was nutrition and metabolism that seemed to excite FDM most. Prior studies looked at the question of how best to spare human protein reserves by the judicious use of essential substrates in various quantities and combinations to gain maximal nitrogen conservation. Not surprisingly, a balanced combination of glucose, fat, glycerol, and amino acids was the most desirable and the most efficacious."[15]

MOORE DESIGNED MANY of his investigations to solve specific clinical problems. Cancer of the breast was a particular interest. In 1894 Halsted introduced the radical mastectomy, a dissection that incorporated the lymphatic drainage and underlying muscles with the breast. Although this procedure became particularly popular in the United States, many of the cancers recurred. The lack of improvement in results, even after half a century, provoked some surgeons in the 1950s and 1960s to re-examine the disease. Investigators began formal and detailed studies of its natural history, the prognostic importance of clinical staging, and the significance of the interval between the original mastectomy and later spread of the tumor. They began to treat local metastases with radiation and to re-consider the influence of the patient's endocrine status.

As a result, operative approaches to change the hormonal milieu in patients with recurrent disease enjoyed a prolonged ascendancy. But while modest objective improvement often lasted for months following removal of the ovaries, clinical investigators soon found that castrated women continued to secrete sex hormones originating in the adrenal glands, stimulated by the pituitary. Indeed, these adrenal estrogens not infrequently enhanced tumor growth.[16] In 1953, surgeons first undertook bilateral adrenalectomy in women with recurrent breast cancer. Removal of the pituitary by Matson and other neurosurgeons also came into vogue. Moore and his group were a driving force behind many of these early studies.

Shortly after his arrival at the Brigham, the new professor established a breast clinic to study patients with the disease and to assess the results of the new treatments alone or in combination. He and his colleagues, particularly Andrew Jessiman and Richard Wilson, followed hundreds of patients over many years, reporting their analyses in a series of influential reviews in the *New England Journal of Medicine*.[17] They described an endocrine assay to determine whether the tumor would respond to the changes in the body's hormonal environment and reviewed the influence of steroids and the differential effects of endocrine ablation. Comparing a large group of patients whose pituitary had been removed to those with adrenalectomy alone, they concluded that the latter procedure was less morbid, as complications were relatively minor, side effects meager, palliation significant, and duration of remission impressive. Indeed, careful case selection produced objective benefit in 60–70% of cases. While chemotherapy was relatively rudimentary at the time, the research group found that particular drugs in combination with adrenalectomy and local radiation were also quite effective. Most importantly, they carefully planned an approach that involved the histology of the cancer, its biological type, its rate of progression, and its reaction to various hormones. These early multimodal strategies, summarized in two sequential departmental monographs, became significant contributions to the evolution of the treatment of breast cancer.

THE ATMOSPHERE IN MOORE'S ever-enlarging department was charged with opportunities for the house staff to become conversant and involved with investigative work, either by reviewing series of cases on particular clinical topics or by spending time in a laboratory. The surgical faculty contributed greatly to the spirit. Under their guidance, many of us became involved in patient-based research projects early in our residencies, learned the art of compiling data, writing medical papers, and occasionally presented our results. Within weeks of the arrival of the new house staff each July, a mimeographed letter from the professor appeared in the mailboxes, entitled *Summer Doldrums*. In it, Moore noted that many in the department would be away during the summer months, often sailing along the coast. As the operative schedule would be relatively light, he suggested that it would be a good idea if interested residents would target a staff mentor and begin a clinical research effort on a subject of mutual interest. I quickly began work with Edward Edwards, for instance, a wise and prolific surgical-anatomist in the department. Collecting patient charts from the record room was easy—all one did was ask the librarian. The records appeared, without fuss, questions, or the need for permission from human subjects committees. I gathered and analyzed the data, published my paper and discussed the findings at a national meeting. Such opportunities stimulated the emergence of many future academic careers.

Ongoing laboratory investigations were discussed at the Tuesday morning research conferences in the surgical library. Moore increased the pressure on potential presenters by arriving early in the hospital the day before and listing on the blackboard what subjects he wanted reviewed. Young research fellows, often for the first time, had to prepare a lecture, make slides, stand before a group, and present their data. The professor sat in the front row of the packed room, inevitably asking relevant questions that penetrated directly to the essential basis of the topic described. New ideas, exposure of experimental flaws, and general discussion ensued. Individuals who had worked in the laboratories or trained at the Brigham still remember those conferences with pleasure, particularly after they learned that the chief would give their particular project undivided attention if they convinced him that he had suggested the topic.

In contrast to many heads of surgical departments in the United States, Moore never insisted that his trainees spend time in research. He did, however, clearly offer the possibilities of joining a laboratory, discussing the point years later. "Every Professor of Surgery who has himself done laboratory research must have a sense of ambivalence on this point. Should every trainee be sent for a period of time in the laboratory? I felt the research was a little like playing the piano. Some people were good at it, and some just were not. There was no use forcing everybody to practice three hours per day. But this view may be too narrow, and maybe it would be better if every young surgeon somehow had an exposure to the laboratory. In some services where this was made a matter of coercion, it resulted only in exploitation and the publication of many worthless papers. Possibly, in the ideally balanced program, each young person could be given an opportunity in the lab and then support it handsomely if his work was promising, or returned to the Clinical Service without prejudice if the laboratory was not a strong point for him."[18]

Those taking the opportunity found that the time spent in research was invaluable, both intellectually and socially. As a result, enthusiastic residents and fellows crowded the laboratories to work with clinical investigators in the hospital or basic scientists at the medical school. Steven Rosenberg was an example of those who continued in the laboratory. Moore allowed him to take several years out of his residency to earn his Ph.D. in immunology. Moving to the National Institutes of Health on completion of his surgical training, his ongoing contributions to the immunologic control of cancer have opened an entirely new field of endeavor. He has directed the National Cancer Institute for many years.

Some residents went to other institutions in the United States. The experience allowed a young doctor, already with several years of clinical training, to think, read, create, and live in other cities for prolonged periods, to interact with unusual personalities, enjoy new areas, and sample different philosophies. Lifelong friends were made.

Others transferred themselves and their families across oceans, and hemispheres. I was one of many of Moore's residents to travel abroad for my research experience. Having become increasingly interested in the mechanisms of rejection and other poorly understood phenomena experienced by the kidney transplant patients I cared for, I spent several years at Oxford University and the University of Glasgow working with some of the foremost cellular immunologists of the time. I immersed myself in my projects, becoming conversant with the field, learning to understand the ability of basic scientists to ask specific questions, design relevant experiments to answer them, and interpret the data. I also found how difficult it is to wrest secrets from Nature! The opportunity changed my entire career.

In like vein, Brennan recalled some of the highlights of his research years, describing well the philosophy of Moore's laboratory. "The laboratory years from 1969–1976 were exciting times. The books had been published, and residents and fellows alike were expected to know each and every one from cover to cover, and to continue to contribute to the further advancement of the metabolic and nutritional care of the surgical patient. Studies continued to examine metabolic responses but they focused predominantly on validation of the methods of determining, particularly with potassium, the consequences of blood transfusion and hemorrhage. We used young volunteers from Harvard Square, usually as a consequence of an advertisement in the *Phoenix* [an 'underground' newspaper], and acutely depleted their red cell mass to a hematocrit of 20, while they were invasively monitored for cardiovascular, pulmonary and peripheral metabolic responses!

"The concept of invasive monitoring is something that would have great trouble getting past any [current] institutional review board. In the early seventies such experimental studies in volunteers seemed to be the norm. When one reviews the published manuscripts, it is interesting to read in the *Materials and Methods* [section] that we took four men and 'although prolonged catheterization of the right heart has not been part of our previous procedures in the study of normal persons, a review of this procedure with a committee of cardiologists indicated it would be a justified procedure, free of hazard.' One wonders how that would be accepted in this day and age. Nevertheless, this was at a time when FDM felt behooved to protect the advances in 'science' from the overzealous restrictions of ethic committees. I well remember his confrontation with the then Review Board Chairman, one of his close friends, 'God damn it—you are getting in the way of scientific progress!' "[19]

This interchange between laboratories and training programs continued for decades, with many of the young investigators later achieving high university positions. Although enhanced by the addition of research workers from Asia in recent years, it should be noted that this felicitous and mutually beneficial arrangement has currently slowed, with fewer American residents entering research because of the changing emphasis in health care, the fact that fewer surgical research laboratories are continuing to function, and lower numbers of foreign applicants seeking positions.

MEMBERS OF THE DEPARTMENT of surgery increased progressively in number during Moore's tenure as an unending influx of research fellows from all over the world worked in his laboratories, attending staff entering new surgical specialties, and residents desiring a place in them were accepted into the program. The professor was a highly visible and

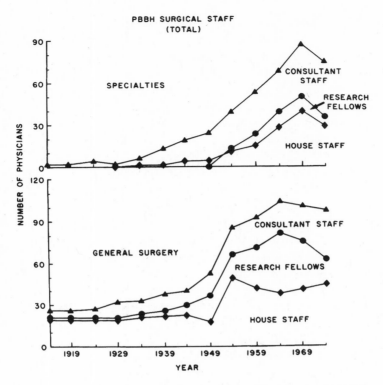

FIGURE 11.4 Changes in numbers of the surgical staff under the three first Brigham surgeons-in-chief.

all-pervasive presence, apparently involved with everything within and outside of surgery. He could speak eloquently on any subject, questioning, cajoling, demanding, and stimulating thought in the operating room, on an individual basis, or leading bedside student and resident rounds, intensive care rounds, morbidity and mortality conferences, and grand rounds. He often presented the results of his laboratory investigations and their clinical relevance at conferences, describing his studies on surgical manpower in the United States, and discussing changes in health care delivery. At the end of these sessions there would inevitably be a pile of his reprints on the subject for the residents to read. Assisting him at operation was an adventure. If things were going well during surgery, he was talkative, ebullient, and inevitably amusing. When they weren't, he became quiet and we could hear traces of asthmatic breathing.

198

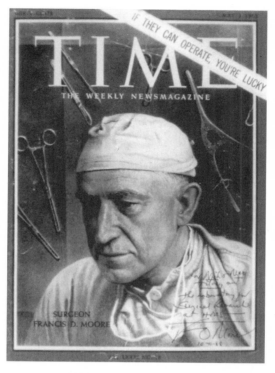

FIGURE 11.5   The cover of *Time* magazine, May 2, 1963
(with permission, Getty Images, Inc.).

In 1969 he initiated a department-wide group practice, the Brigham Surgical Group. This venture, the first at a Harvard institution, pooled resources to support young faculty and researchers and to improve retirement benefits for the staff. Such was its effectiveness that many other teaching hospitals throughout the country copied the plan. He became president of major professional societies, was active on national committees, and was widely sought as a lecturer throughout the world. He spent much time commuting to Washington D.C. as a consultant to the Army and to NASA, as a member of NIH study sections, and as a force in planning the Uniformed Services University. An enthusiastic sailor, he papered the walls of the surgeons' lounge with charts of the New England coast. I remember once making my way across the street to the surgical laboratory in the medical school where he had invited all his research personnel and anyone else interested to hear about his cruise back from Bermuda following The Race. The talk comprised a series of slides showing mostly waves and occasional gulls. Several days worth. But he even presented this in an exciting manner. The large audience filling the laboratory loved it.

Moore vigorously pursued a variety of interests in health care policy throughout his career. During the late 1960s, he had become heavily involved with a labor organizer and the dean of Harvard Medical School in establishing an "academic based, non-profit, pre-paid health delivery plan," later termed a health maintenance organization (HMO).[20] One of the earliest such schemes in the United States, Harvard Community Health Plan (HCHP) prospered for many years, delivering excellent care by university-based surgeons and physicians. "Our hospital was asked to make available all our residents and emergency staffing (without extra pay) for the subscribers to HCHP." In contrast to many other insurance schemes evolving at the time, however, both Moore and George Thorn insisted that all segments of society should benefit, including minority residents in the neighborhood who could not pay for treatment. Federal agencies sponsoring health care financing for the poor, particularly the Office of Economic Opportunity, underwrote the broad coverage. Gordon Vineyard, a long-time member of the department, became director of surgery for the rapidly enlarging plan. But like so many other HMO's in the current era, it ultimately began to lose its inclusivity and non-profit status with increasingly restrictive constraints on membership. This often-inadequate pattern of health care delivery remains unresolved.

As the professor grew older, he became increasingly outspoken about the problem of corporate profits in the health care budget in the United States, decrying as medical "profiteering" the often-huge hospital surpluses and the excessive incomes of some doctors. As late as 1997, he and his influential co-author, John McArthur, the Dean of the Harvard Business School, called for reform in a frequently quoted paper. "The current trend toward the invasion of commerce into medical care, an arena formally under the exclusive purvue of physicians, is seen by the authors as an epic clash of cultures between commercial and professional traditions in the United States. Both have contributed to society for centuries, and both have much to offer in strengthening medical care and reducing costs. At the same time, this invasion by commercialism of an area formally governed by professionalism poses

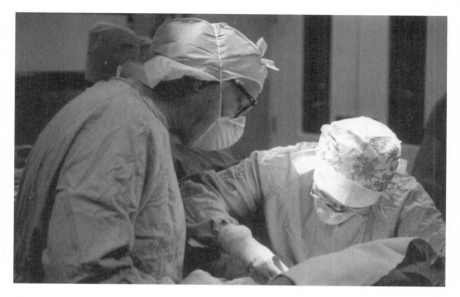

FIGURE 11.6   Moore operating with the first female surgical resident, Robin Goodfellow, 1974.

severe hazards to the care of the sick and the welfare of communities: the health of the public and the public health."[21]

Like Cushing and Cutler before him, Moore spent much effort considering the role of the surgeon-scientist, the training of the surgeon, and the quality of surgical care. A product of his time, he did not accept a woman or member of a minority group into the residency until the early 1970s. Most of us in the department felt that this was not a considered omission but that such a departure had never occurred to him despite mounting societal pressures in the United States during that period.

He extended much effort on the question of surgical manpower, becoming a co-director of a large national effort to re-examine the current status of surgery. Ultimately sponsored both by the American Surgical Association and the American College of Surgeons, the *Study on Surgical Services for the United States* (*SOSSUS*) examined several aspects of the profession, particularly the over-supply and under-employment of surgeons.[22] After he and his committee gathered and analyzed large amounts of data, they recommended that numbers of surgical trainees should be reduced and credentialing standards raised by appropriate professional bodies to balance the increased numbers of young surgeons looking for positions.

Part of their conclusions on control of residency size and quality involved foreign medical graduates. Those from highly developed countries entering excellent training programs enhanced surgery in the United States. In contrast, many from under-developed countries often joined relatively weak training programs. If they stayed, their inferior surgical education lowered the standard of care; if they returned to their own countries they found they were inadequately prepared. Indeed, during the 1970s the percentage of foreign graduates in various training programs ranged from a low of 7% in neurosurgery to a high of 35% in colorectal and thoracic surgery.

But despite the completeness and accuracy of *SOSSUS*, many surgeons and their professional organizations greeted the results and conclusions with predictable animosity. Moore and others persisted, however, in producing status reports on accredited surgical manpower in the United States over the next two decades. The data led to continuing reforms.

As one of the foremost surgical-scientists of his time and a significant figure in international surgery, Moore evoked awe and probably fear among his house staff. He would meet with each of us once a year, inquiring about our careers, our goals, and our families. We all felt flattered by the gesture. "For those of us who were privileged to be residents in his program, I never went to a meeting where, if at least two Brigham residents were present, he was not discussed! We all admired, respected, revered, and indeed, loved him, although love would not be something he uniformly reciprocated for the residents! He was much too concerned about ensuring that they excelled, that they moved ahead, and that they made a difference. I expect he liked the residents, but he also expected much of them. I never saw him criticize. The frequent implication was, 'you can do better.' "[23] Many of his trainees did!

CHAPTER 12

DIGITS AND DEVICES

DESPITE THE SUCCESSES that Gross, Blalock, and others had achieved in treating congenital defects of the heart and great vessels in children, realistic expectations for the surgical correction of acquired cardiac disease in adults did not ripen until after World War II. One spark that ignited the new interest was a report by Dwight Harken describing the successful removal of foreign bodies from in and around the hearts of wounded soldiers.

Harken had interned at Bellevue Hospital in New York City after Harvard Medical School, then trained in London with Tudor Edwards, one of the foremost thoracic surgeons of the time. While learning the newest techniques of lung and esophageal surgery, he became increasingly intrigued by the possibilities of operating on the human heart despite the long-enduring sentiments of the surgical establishment against such a step. As bacterial endocarditis was a relatively common and inevitably fatal condition in that pre-antibiotic era, Harken had initiated a series of clinically applicable studies in dogs aimed at clearing vegetations from the surface of infected mitral valves via the left atrium.

Posted to an Army hospital in England during the war and faced with severe combat injuries, he dedicated his energies to treating wounds of the chest and later reported his experience in removing bullets and other bits of shrapnel from 134 soldiers without a fatality.[1] These included 78 missiles from the great vessels and 56 involving the heart itself. He extracted 13 of these from inside the cardiac chambers, using the methods he had perfected in experimental animals. Although French and British surgeons had excised bullets close to the hearts of a handful of the wounded in World War I, Harken's large and successful clinical series was unprecedented.

He was faced initially with a soldier badly injured during the D-day landings. An x-ray showed a metallic foreign body lodged in the heart.

Quickly opening the chest, he discovered that the foreign body lay within the right ventricle. He described the subsequent events in a letter to his wife. "For a moment, I stood with my clamp on the fragment that was inside the heart, and the heart was not bleeding. Then suddenly, with a pop as if a champagne cork had been drawn, the fragment jumped out of the ventricle, forced by the pressure within the chamber. Blood poured out in a torrent." Tightening the superficial sutures he had placed around the defect was ineffectual. "I [then] told the assistants to cross the sutures and I put my fingers over the awful leak. The torrent slowed, stopped, and with my finger *in situ*, I took large needles swedged with silk and began passing them through the heart muscle wall, under my finger, and out the other side. With four of these in, I slowly removed my finger as one after the other was tied. Blood pressure did drop, but the only moment of panic was when we discovered that one suture had gone through the glove on the finger that had stemmed the flood. I was sutured to the wall of the heart! We cut the glove and I got loose."[2] The patient recovered.

In 1948 Moore invited Harken, a flamboyant and optimistic figure, to join the Brigham staff as chief of thoracic and cardiac surgery. During the three years he had spent at the Boston City Hospital immediately following the conflict, he had become increasingly interested in the tragic problems posed by mitral stenosis and attracted to the possibilities of opening the valve surgically to treat those afflicted. This common and often life-threatening condition occurred in relatively young patients who had developed rheumatic fever following an earlier streptococcal infection, the course of which could not be influenced, as penicillin was not yet available. Evaluating some of the physiological consequences of the narrowed valve in laboratory animals, he confirmed that its hemodynamic effects included pulmonary hypertension and progressive myocardial dysfunction. Arrhythmias allowed clots to form in the dilated left atrium; these often migrated as arterial emboli to brain, bowel, or lower extremities.

The possibility of curing those afflicted by opening the valve surgically was attractive. Although Sir Lauder Brunton had originally identified the need for corrective operation early in the century, no one had subsequently considered such a step except Cutler, who had successfully opened the valves of a young patient via the ventricle in 1923, and Sir Henry Souttar at the London Hospital, who had felt a mitral valve in a single individual by placing his finger through the left atrial appendage in 1925. Souttar later wrote to Harken that "I did not repeat the operation because I could not get another case. Although my patient made an uninterrupted recovery the Physicians declared that it was all nonsense and that the operation was unjustified. It is of no use to be ahead of one's time."[3]

As another example of different investigators in different locations and unbeknownst to each other arriving at the same idea at the same time, three surgeons began to operate on stenotic mitral valves virtually simultaneously in the late 1940s. In Philadelphia, Charles Bailey first used a dilator to open the valves of four patients. All died. At the Boston City Hospital, Harken abortively introduced Cutler's valvulotome into the mitral valve of his first patient through the left superior pulmonary vein, describing the unsuccessful result to him (Cutler) on his deathbed. His first success with his "valvuloplasty" occurred in his second attempt on June 16, 1948, just six days after Bailey's first successful "commissurotomy." "I felt this (16 June surgery) was so important and should be published promptly so I rushed to Joe Garland, Editor of the *New England Journal of Medicine*, and told him to get it published as quickly as possible. He did and it was published November 1948. Actually, again Charlie [Bailey] scooped me for he published in the *Chicago Daily News* or some similar Chicago paper."[4] And within a few months, Russell Brock in London reintroduced Souttar's technique, opening the valves of eight patients with his finger inserted through the left atrial appendage. Six survived. His effective use of the finger fracture method quickly convinced the others. But patients continued to die regardless of the approach. Harken wrote a rather bleak report of his first five attempts "only to indicate the ability of such patients to withstand the operation. The evaluation of any long-term benefits attributed to this procedure must rest on objective criteria gained from [then minimal or nonexistent] hemodynamic studies."[5]

Despite the support of occasional visionaries enthusiastic about the possibilities of cardiac surgery, patient mortality from the mitral operations did not improve appreciably for several years. Indeed, most surgeons remained skeptical about the value of the procedure. At the Brigham the results were so bleak that the surgical residents petitioned Moore to halt the program. Pressure from colleagues to wait for new developments was also strong. John Gibbon, a surgeon at the MGH working on a heart-lung apparatus "urged a moratorium on surgical intervention until his cardiopulmonary bypass could render direct

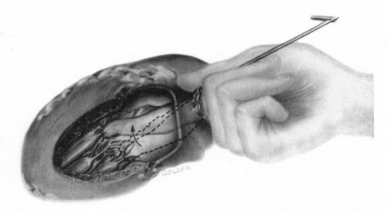

FIGURE 12.1   Harken's technique of opening the mitral valve digitally via the transatrial approach.

vision surgery available, an innovation which he felt to be on the verge of practical realization."[6] But regardless of these and other blandishments, Harken and occasionally other interested surgeons persisted "with the confidence inspired by the substantial palliation accomplished by 'finger fracture' and valvulotome valvuloplasty in patients with pure mitral stenosis." Increasingly enamored with the digital procedure, he characteristically had the operating nurse cut the finger off his rubber glove before he entered the beating heart via the left atrial appendage. He had "a specially prepared fingernail grown long then trimmed in offset fashion similar to the blade of a carpenter's knife. Furthermore, tiny notches were cut into the free edge, converting the nail into a miniature saw." Even in those dismal early days when so many died, Moore encouraged Harken to continue, as he believed the operation to be a good one with important future possibilities.

The numbers of patients grew exponentially. In 1959, Harken and a cardiologic colleague, Laurence Ellis, reported the results of 1000 mitral valvuloplasties.[7] While the initial results were disappointing, the progressive improvement was remarkable. The early mortality for the first 100 patients was 32% for the sickest and 14% for the most favorable. For patients 101 to 500, the death rate fell to 24% and 4%, respectively. For numbers 501 to 1,000, it declined to 20% and 0.6%, respectively. In 1973 they published a 15–20 year follow-up on these individuals, a unique clinical experience.[8] The efficacy of operative relief of mitral stenosis, as they described in their reports, was critical

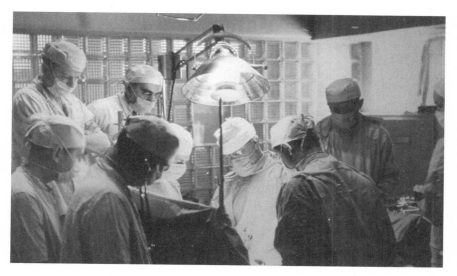

Figure 12.2   Harken and his team performing an early mitral commissurotomy.

to the convictions of a growing body of medical and surgical investigators that operative correction of lesions of heart valves was a realistic choice for seriously ill patients.

As bold in diagnosing of cardiac abnormalities as Harken was in performing heart surgery, Lewis Dexter became a close collaborator in many of the ongoing advances. An innovative cardiovascular physiologist, he had joined the department of medicine at the Brigham in 1941. His initial studies of hypertension led him to sample levels of the hormone, renin, from the renal veins via a venous catheter. Late in 1944 he carried out, by serendipity, one of the first catheterizations of the right side of the human heart. He recalled the incident. "I decided to wander around the heart which I understood was above the diaphragm somewhere. Suddenly, the catheter came clear out in the lung field and I was sure I [had] perforated the heart. I didn't have any idea what to do and I turned on the overhead lights and said, 'Mr. S—, how are you?' He said, 'I feel a hell of a lot better than you look.' Then I was pretty sure that, having perforated the heart it just sort of sealed itself off. So I closed my eyes and then I pulled the catheter back and nothing happened. I went and looked up the anatomy of the chest and I figured I had gone into the pulmonary artery."[9]

Hearing of his adventure later that day, the dean of the medical school suggested that if Dexter could routinely place a catheter into the pulmonary artery, he would be able to examine various heart diseases in detail. He was able and his subsequent studies defined a variety of hemodynamic abnormalities occurring with congenital heart defects. He also soon discovered that the pulmonary capillary wedge pressure (wedging the catheter tip deep into a small branch of the pulmonary artery) was an accurate measure of left atrial and left ventricular filling pressures, critical in determining the extent of valvular abnormalities.

Dexter was also the first to show that exercise with a cardiac catheter in place in the right heart was safe and could provide clinically significant data. "[He] did not believe that he should subject anybody to a procedure that he himself would not be willing to undergo. He asked one of his fellows to place a catheter in his [Dexter's] pulmonary artery. Once the catheter was in, [he] gently sat up and then very gently dangled his feet. Everyone was watching and everyone was frightened. Was he going to have a cardiac arrest? (Remember this was before the invention of defibrillators.) And then he stood up. Then he started to skip a little, and then proceeded to do vigorous exercise. He promptly recorded all the responses before removing the catheter."[10]

Interest in the treatment of patients with acquired disease of their cardiac valves was a natural progression of these studies, stimulated further by Harken's surgical activity. Using the new techniques of left heart catheterization, Dexter and his junior associate, Richard Gorlin, examined the significance of mitral valve gradients and determined the critical size of a given stenotic orifice that required surgical intervention. Along with investigators at other centers, they tested several methods to determine left atrial pressure, including transbronchial and transesophageal puncture techniques.[11] They then extended the scanty knowledge of the pathophysiology of aortic stenosis by measuring cardiac output using dye dilution curves. First using a needle, then introducing a polyethylene catheter through the left atrium into the left ventricle, they quantified the flow across the affected valves of patients with "pure" aortic stenosis, calculating the cross-sectional area and defining better criteria for operative repair. Gorlin soon developed a formula to determine the orifice size of stenotic valves and introduced cardiac angiography to the Brigham. About the same time, Dexter established one of the original research cardiac catheterization laboratories. A colleague, Bernard Lown, opened an early cardiac care unit.

With the increasing availability of the respirator and a variety of monitoring devices, Harken then initiated the first postoperative intensive care unit (ICU) for cardiac surgical patients, a concept rapidly extended to include ICUs for acute medical and surgical illnesses. Patients with heart disease were receiving increasing attention by those concentrating exclusively on their problems.

With data accumulating on the circulatory abnormalities of valvular disease, Harken and his cardiologist colleagues broadened their treatment plans. Patients with stenosis of the tricuspid and mitral valves provided the next challenge as they realized that expected improvement might not occur unless both valves were opened. Acknowledging a technique described previously by others, they refined an operative approach for simultaneous repair of both valves through a single left thoracotomy incision.[12]

As the results of the procedure were promising, they began to consider comparable ways to relieve aortic stenosis. As the blind, uncontrolled technique of transventricular aortic valve fracture led to an immediate operative mortality of over 20%, Harken attempted to fracture the valve by placing his finger through an operating tunnel of a synthetic material sewn onto the ascending aorta, but reported 16 operative deaths and 12 late deaths in a series of a 100 patients.[13] With these poor results as background, he and his colleagues examined systematically the hemodynamic significance and natural history of the condition, assessing the life expectancy of those with the disease and characterizing the ominous significance of left ventricular failure as manifested by shortness of breath. Based on increasing data from the cardiac laboratory, they formulated surgical indications for its correction. At the same time, other surgeons were addressing the problem using methods that included a transventricular approach to dilate the valve, open operations to remove calcium directly from the leaflets, or tailoring or reconstructing abnormal leaflets with the heart stopped under hypothermia. Most of these approaches were ineffectual.

The need for a mechanical device to replace an irrevocably damaged valve was obvious. As accurate placement of any substitute required a still heart in a bloodless field, those contemplating such definitive operations had to have a means to stop ventricular function while maintaining normal circulation of oxygenated blood to the rest of the body. The answer was an external cardiopulmonary bypass connected to the patient via a major artery and vein.

Using such a device in 1953, John Gibbon successfully closed an intra-atrial septal defect in the stopped heart of an 18-year-old girl, a feat he was never able to repeat.[14] She had been supported on bypass for 26 minutes. Despite a prevailing sense of pessimism among his colleagues toward the future of the enterprise, he had single-mindedly collaborated with his wife for two decades in developing the pump-oxygenator, first at the MGH and then at Jefferson University.

Francis Moore recalls amusingly a visit to Gibbon's laboratory in Philadelphia to see how "the Great Machine was coming along. We trooped in, 10 or 15 of us, and were asked to take off our shoes and put on rubber boots. We were then ushered into the operating room. At that time the pump oxygenator was approximately the size of a grand piano. A small cat, asleep on one side, was the object of all this attention. The cat was connected to the machine by two transparent blood filled plastic tubes. The contrast in size between the small cat and the huge machine aroused considerable amusement among the audience. Watching this complicated procedure, concentrating mostly on the cat, whose heart was about to be completely isolated from its circulation, opened, and then closed, we began to sense that we were not walking on a dry floor. We looked down. We were standing in an inch of blood. 'Oh, I'm sorry' said Gibbon 'the confounded thing has sprung a leak again,' but his machine opened an entirely new era in surgery."[15]

While the concept was clear, much of Gibbon's research involved identifying the most effective materials for the apparatus (at the beginning of his experiments, only gum rubber tubing was available; the existing glass or metal connections or cannulae promoted clotting), devising means to decrease the threat of air embolism from bubbles in the system, constructing effective pumps and valves, instituting ways to control volume, pressure, flow, and temperature, and designing satisfactory methods to oxygenate blood. By the early 1950s, evolving improvements allowed prolonged (up to 46 minutes) extracorporeal support of dogs and cats. Gibbon's first patient was a 15 month old, operated on in February 1952 to repair a large atrial septal defect. Unfortunately, without the availability of cardiac catheterization, the diagnosis was incorrect. At autopsy, she was found to have a large, unrecognized patent ductus arteriosus. His second and final attempt a year later was successful.

Encouraged by this case, surgical teams in the United States and Europe built a series of cardiopulmonary bypass apparatuses and began to test them in patients. Harken too was active in this new enterprise, designing prototypes of bubble, reverse incline plane, concentric bubble, and centrifuge oxygenators. While some of these were produced commercially, they never became popular, as designs from other laboratories proved more effective.

Open heart surgery was a daunting prospect for the residents during that period. The night before the operation, we filled out requisitions for 18 units of blood both to prime the pump and to replace the blood loss expected during the procedure. The circuitry of tubing connecting the patient to the apparatus was also so complex that few of us understood it. Not infrequently, clamps placed on the wrong segment during the initiation of bypass would result in an explosion of blood from the machine that quickly covered the floor. Harken, ever dramatic, would raise his eyes heavenward and emote, "Is here no one here who can help me!" But with progressive improvements in the developing technology, direct valve replacement and repair of other cardiac abnormalities became increasingly possible.

On March 10th, 1960, Harken was the first surgeon ever to place a caged ball prosthesis into the subcoronary position in a patient with aortic insufficiency.[16] The relative success of the Hufnagel ball valve in correcting the condition had stimulated others to use extrinsic baffles

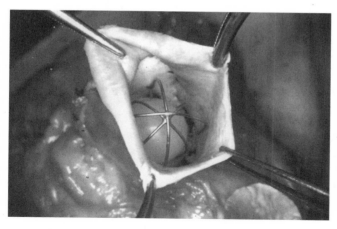

Figure 12.3   Harken's aortic ball valve and its Ivalon baffle in place in the subcoronary position, 1962.

211

to narrow the base of the aorta or repair the valve cusps directly. Several groups, including Harken and his research fellows, had initiated extensive laboratory studies to determine pulse contour, hydraulic and hemodynamic effectiveness of various ball valves and to assess their proper shape and dimensions to fit into the aortic root.[17] Materials for the ball were tested for fatigue, durability, resistance of flow, and trauma to formed blood elements. I well remember going to the Surgical Research Laboratory during this period to be greeted by a cacophony of clicking noises from a variety of ball valve prototypes being tested for long-term function and wear. Operative techniques for their insertion were devised in dogs, all made possible by increasingly effective cardiopulmonary bypass devices. Although the first to be used in a patient, Harken's valve was bulky and difficult to place. A superior device, designed by Albert Starr and Lowell Edwards at the University of Oregon, soon became the valve of choice.[18]

Harken's contributions and innovations continued to mount into "a series of pioneering ventures with a record of accomplishments so numerous and significant that he is often considered one of the fathers of heart surgery."[19] His innovations included the development of the direct current (DC) defibrillator, and the concept of counter pulsation which led to the development of the intra-aortic balloon pump to sustain those in heart failure.[20] He and his group designed, produced, and installed the first demand pacemaker in 1966. "Testing was exhaustive against every conceivable electrical interference. However, [Ralph] Nader's group [later] chastised me at a congressional hearing for not testing against the microwave oven! (The microwave oven hit the market *in 1967*—a little tough to test in 1966!)."[21]

AS MORE COMPREHENSIVE and accurate technologies to monitor complex post-operative patients were emerging, more specialized units were becoming necessary for support of the seriously ill. While a recovery room existed adjacent to the operating rooms, it was too small to accommodate Harken's ever-increasing numbers of cardiac patients, Murray's transplant recipients, and individuals on Moore's service with severe burns and metabolic complications. Alfred Morgan, a staff surgeon heavily involved with the care and study of the latter cases, recalls the first ICU opening in 1960, as "a 3-bed space behind the main recovery room which had been variously a corridor to the Anesthesia Department offices, a place to store ventilators, and a recovery area for post-operative cardiac patients. At one time we kept them for days when too sick to discharge sooner. One stayed in OR 5 for a month."[22]

Moore had already put aside an area designed for the study and treatment of seriously ill patients, modeled after Fuller Albright's Ward 4 at the MGH. The nurses were trained specifically to measure everything the patients took in and put out. Albright's precise metabolic charts acted as templates for Moore's own standardized documentation of physiologic changes. Morgan continues: "There was an assumption that the most significant problems were associated with the sickest people, so the Bartlett Unit became a de-facto ICU. No one knew then what an ICU was supposed to look like anyhow but it was plain that to put sick people in a room at the end of a corridor and close the door was undesirable. This was one reason for our interest in monitoring. It was electronic babysitting, using technology and organization to overcome inappropriate architecture."

Always an original thinker, the new professor was a master at recognizing the importance of novel concepts and trends to improve patient care. He pursued strenuously the idea of an ICU and a clinical research center when few other hospitals had done so. He was one of the first to introduce computerized information gathering in surgery, later testing a computer controlled transfusion model as an algorithm for accurate maintenance of various hemodynamic parameters after heart surgery. Data generated by the computer clearly outpaced those produced by the residents. Morgan noted further that "things came together to make intensive care take off like a rocket. The climate was just right. Attitudes were favorable. There was an appreciation for the complex (lots of people in medicine then still wanted simple solutions for everything), and an openness to novelty and serendipity." Indeed, the professor displayed a homily conspicuously in the research conference room for all to contemplate: "You find only what you look for. You look for only what you know."

Moore deliberately collected a multi-disciplined coterie of young faculty to work in the new areas, as illustrated in a letter he sent to Morgan. "I am writing you this note to outline the position which we are offering you upon completion of your residency. As we have discussed in our previous conversations, I want you to come here and join us with your primary orientation towards the intensive care of the critically ill patient. Your particular contribution in this field will at least initially lie in the aspects of instrumentation, measurement, monitoring, presentation, collection and analysis of data. You will be joining a team effort that involves both general surgery and anesthesia. You will be in a sense be the center man of this team, helping us to develop more adequate methods for monitoring and measuring the events of these patients. [Members of the team include those] interested in biochemical aspects, particularly the peripheral chemical indices of low flow states, inhalation therapy, [and] the measurement of ventilation, ventilatory adequacy, and ventilation:perfusion ratios.

The specifics of the position were less sanguine. "It will be our object to give you a Brigham appointment as Junior Associate and a Harvard appointment as either Instructor or Assistant. We would like to arrange a salary for you in the region of $11,000–$12,000 per year. This money would come in part from research grants, in part from the hospital, in part from other funds, and possibly in part from the university budget."[23] As many of us can attest, the financial comfort of his staff was never one of his primary considerations.

Monitor, collect, and analyze they did. "We [John Collins, Harken's eventual successor, was another principal in the project working with Morgan. He had supplemented his general surgical residency at the Brigham by training with a pioneer in cardiac surgery at the University of Alabama, John Kirklin.] were greedy for information, so for a time patient data were recorded on multi channel reel to reel data channel recorders. Physiology's tools were moving to bedside medicine and we began measuring and recording endovascular pressures, beat to beat and breath-to-breath vital signs, and doing frequent indicator dilution cardiac outputs. Several projects in this cluster were aimed at making measurement easier or more nearly continuous. Pretty soon we had more monitoring data than we could deal with. One of Kirklin's engineers noted that we needed a computer. He already had one, a refrigerator-sized IBM machine. He had configured it to log hemodynamic data and use the information to control blood infusion after heart surgery and it worked. We [Morgan and Collins] found the Hewlett Packard Corporation interested. [They made] microcomputers sized like microwave ovens."

The monitored ICU patients arranged themselves into predictable categories. "Balance patients had everything going in and coming out collected, sampled, and analyzed. Usually there were one or more patients with major burns studied both for changes in body composition and for the dynamics of surface bacteriology. Brigham surgeons quickly described what later was to be termed 'multiple system failure' in another frequent type, the POGARF, an acronym [coined by a surgical resident] that stood for 'post-operative grief with acute renal failure.' "[24] Care of such individuals involved intermittent hemodialysis, a relatively unique form of treatment not in routine use in many centers at the time. Fasting humans, all obese and all volunteers, were studied in detail, sometimes for many months. Morgan remembers this population "as a natural application for isotope dilution [for] measurement of body composition that also had obvious relevance to surgical topics. To know how the body conserves itself in fasting should help understand how conservation fails in trauma and sepsis." Data for scientific papers, presentations at conferences, and major addresses flowed from these patients.

As a Brigham surgical resident during the 1960s, Robert Bartlett was well aware of the new ideas and technologies that were beginning to influence the care of the seriously ill. Developing an enduring interest in respiratory failure during his rotation at Children's Hospital, he realized that children developing pulmonary dysfunction following prolonged operations for complex congenital cardiac defects could eventually recover if they remained alive during the post-operative period. He queried Robert Gross whether "we could use the heart-

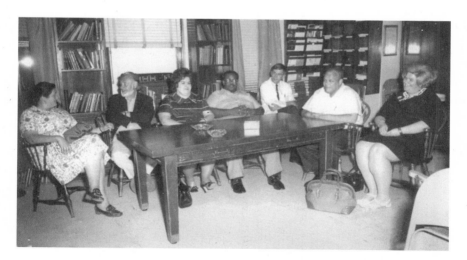

FIGURE 12.4   Alfred Morgan and patients volunteering for the obesity study.

215

lung machine for a few days to sustain the life of these patients until their native hearts recovered. He observed that the heart-lung machine was itself a lethal instrument if used for more than an hour or two, but he encouraged our research to extend [its] use for longer periods of time."[25] This exchange may have triggered Bartlett's interest in membrane oxygenation to support patients with severe pulmonary insufficiency.

At the same time, care of adult patients who developed this syndrome had become a major research interest of the Brigham department. "Post-traumatic Pulmonary Insufficiency" was an increasingly common condition that developed after severe injury or extensive surgery. It was characterized by atelectasis, poor compliance, leakage from pulmonary capillaries, transpulmonary shunting of blood, and increasing pulmonary vascular resistance. In 1965 Moore hired Philip Drinker, an engineer from MIT, to consider the increasingly obvious need for artificial ventilation to support those afflicted.

As Drinker's father had been one of the inventors of the "iron lung" for polio victims in the 1930s, he was familiar with the task. He

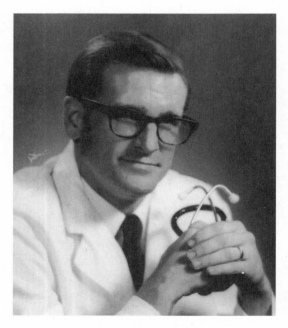

FIGURE 12.5   Robert Bartlett.

216

describes the background. "It had become clear that the population of respiratory care patients was changing markedly. Rather than the polio victim with essentially normal lungs, a new group of patients was emerging who showed acute respiratory dysfunction, frequently following major trauma not involving the thorax—patients who earlier would never have survived long enough to reach the ICU. The understanding, prevention, and care of this new type of respiratory lesion—known variously as post-traumatic pulmonary insufficiency, acute respiratory distress syndrome (ARDS), or obliterative pneumonitis—formed the focus of most of the respiratory research during the 1960s at the Brigham as at other centers. The threat of polio had nearly vanished in the previous decade.

"Great strides had been made in positive pressure ventilation, a novel technique introduced largely during the last great polio epidemic in Scandinavia when they ran out of iron lungs. Antibiotics allowed safer and more stable management of tracheostomies. The general availability of reliable blood gas machines (the Brigham got its first one in 1960), ventilators of several types, and transducers, amplifiers, oscilloscopes and flow directed catheters set the stage for a sophisticated level of intensive care that demanded education or re-education in basic physiology. In the decade of the 1960s, these measurements became available to every physician, and in the 1970s it was considered malpractice to ignore the advances. But not all the changes were positive. With the end of polio, many respiratory care units closed; when ventilatory support was needed it was usually provided on the general floors. The practice at the time (in many hospitals) was to change the red rubber suction catheter once daily, rinsing after use, and soaking in murky alcohol, also changed once a day. When the surgical ICU opened at the Brigham, it was some years before a dependable supply of disposable sterile suction catheters became available."[26]

A result of this sustained departmental effort was the publication of the book *Post-Traumatic Pulmonary Insufficiency*.[27] This quickly became the standard text in the field. A review suggested its uniqueness and importance. "The purpose of this slim volume is to look beyond clinical platitudes and to define the terminal mechanism that makes lethal injuries lethal. The problem is stated thus: 'When an injured person is resuscitated from a low flow state and dies a week later in intensive care with progressive anoxic coma under oxygen treatment, conventional means to describe this death are often meaningless.' With Moorelike energy, the authors have rearranged and synthesized a syndrome out of the 'meaningless.' "[28]

Time limitations in the use of cardiopulmonary bypass in heart surgery were becoming increasingly obvious during this early period, with clotting, bleeding disorders, edema, and declining organ function not infrequently developing after a few hours of continuous use.[29] As many of these changes resulted from direct exposure of blood to oxygen, Bartlett and Drinker realized that an "artificial lung" with a permeable membrane interposed between blood and gas was needed to sustain afflicted patients for periods often lasting several days. "Laboratory research began on prolonged extracorporeal circulation by those studying function and improvement of membrane lungs."[30] The investigators were also aware that oxygen was overused and that its administration at high concentrations and for prolonged periods was toxic.

Drinker recalled one conversation. "One morning during ICU rounds, the topic came up, and the discussion arose about using a bank of cylinders of different O_2 mixtures, but this seemed a cumbersome solution at best. A bedside air-O2 mixer presented an attractive alternative, although a certain amount of skepticism was expressed initially. A working prototype was tried in patients in the intensive care unit, the first practical gas blender for use with ventilators. The entire project, from conception to clinical application, took about seven months, moving slowly without benefit of oversight by a Human Subjects Committee." Indeed, Bartlett, Drinker, and their collaborators *were* the Human Subject Committee!

Although a membrane oxygenator had been available since the mid-1960s as an alternative to the existing bubble and disk devices, the oxygenator component of the apparatus still limited its effectiveness. Despite adequate gas exchange, plasma proteins denatured, red cells hemolysed and platelets and leukocytes clumped to block capillary flow. Tiny air bubbles formed in the circulating blood. Clotting disorders ensued. While less traumatic to the blood elements, they were "bulky, leaky and undesirable."

Drinker addressed the problem by designing a torus, a circular blood-membrane container rotating on an eccentric axis. Refined from an earlier model, injury to blood was significantly reduced and the oxygen transfer rate of the newly available, thin silicone membrane highly efficient. "Flushed with success, we presented the work at one of Dr. Moore's Tuesday morning research seminars. It was well received and led to many discussions, of which a particularly enjoyable one with Dr. Harken took place in the Cutler lounge. With his typically enthusiastic outlook, he wanted us to apply it clinically right away. We pointed out that the device was still in a very primitive state, and that there were many aspects of it that we wanted to study and analyze. His response, probably heard at the far end of the OR: 'Analyze, hell, we can test it!' "

The investigators used their membrane oxygenator in awake dogs over five-day periods. All physical signs and laboratory tests remained normal. Minimal heparinization during the procedure did not affect blood clotting; only occasionally were small emboli found in the lungs after a week. They also noted that the physiologic responses to the prolonged perfusion, assessed in many experimental subjects, were quite different from the profound changes following cardiopulmonary bypass. Continuous improvement of the apparatus over the next few years made it ready for clinical use. Bartlett recalled that their successes were "common enough nowadays, but pretty exciting stuff in 1966."

Other laboratories began to confirm their findings. A team in California first used Extracorporeal Membrane Oxygenation (ECMO), as

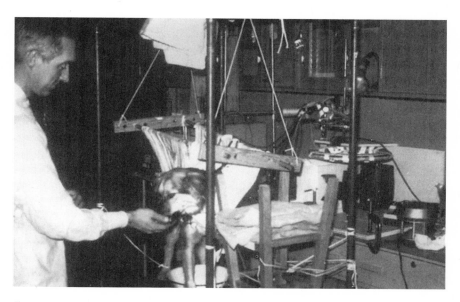

Figure 12.6 Philip Drinker and a dog sustained by ECMO for a week.

the technique was named, successfully in a patient in 1971.[31] Bartlett, who had moved to another university, treated a child in cardiogenic shock the next year.[32] She also survived. Drinker and his colleagues at the Brigham then placed an individual dying with respiratory insufficiency on their oxygenator, a 33-year-old woman who had developed recurrent glomerulonephritis in her kidney isograft. An associated antibody response produced massive bleeding into her lungs. Oxygenation declined dangerously. She became hypotensive. Thirteen hours after an emergency transplant nephrectomy performed in the ICU, ECMO was started and continued for 90 hours. She recovered quickly thereafter and lived on chronic dialysis for years.[33]

Since these early experiences, the use of the "artificial lung" has saved the lives of many children and adults, as Bartlett recently confirmed in a review of his experience with the first 1000 cases, alone or in conjunction with other machines to support failing hearts and kidneys or as a bridge to transplantation.[34] At the same time, he and his colleagues went on to examine the influence of parenteral nutrition ("the artificial gut") on critically ill patients with multiple organ failure, crediting a lesson learned as a resident that adequate carbohydrate and protein supplements may reverse deficient calories and negative nitrogen balance in the critically ill. Indeed, they noted that 90% of individuals in positive caloric balance during their ICU stay survived, but only 20% of those with a profound caloric deficit.[35]

He summarized the overall experience, echoing the teachings of Moore and all others who have worked in applied investigations in surgery. "As in any other combined laboratory and clinical research endeavor, the spinoff from our research has been much more exciting and interesting than the original problem. We have learned a lot about the pathophysiology of critical illness, bioengineering, basic science, the technology of extracorporeal circulation, mechanical ventilation and lung healing. One example of this spinoff is the most difficult step in translating basic research to clinical practice: methods to study life support devices in prospective randomized trials in which the end point is death and the control group [received] conventional treatment."[36]

CHAPTER 13

KIDNEY TRANSPLANTATION
AND THE NOBEL PRIZE

A GAINST THE ADVICE of colleagues in the department, Joseph Murray transplanted a kidney between identical twins on December 23, 1954. Considering the uremic recipient too unstable for general anesthesia, Vandam administered a spinal, an infrequently used technique. Harrison removed the kidney from the etherized donor in an adjacent operating room. Murray placed it in a retro-peritoneal pouch in the lower abdomen, an approach he had perfected in the laboratory and in the autopsy room. After he revascularized the graft and Harrison implanted the ureter directly into the bladder, it began to excrete large amounts of urine. The patient improved rapidly as renal function stabilized. His enlarged heart decreased in size, metabolic abnormalities disappeared, and high blood pressure diminished. Over the next few days, however, he developed a rapid heartbeat and positive urine cultures. Hypertension recurred. Realizing that the diseased native organs were probably responsible for these complications, the surgical team removed them sequentially, a radical maneuver at the time. Recovery thereafter was striking.

The first hurdle faced by the clinical team in preparing for the operation was to prove that the patient and his brother were truly identical. In addition to blood typing and confirmation of various physical characteristics, the workup included exchange of skin grafts. Nothing suggested that donor and recipient were genetically dissimilar. While those involved had not publicly discussed the case, the media's discovery of the proposed procedure began when the police fingerprinted the two brothers as a supplemental means to detect differences. A reporter assigned to the police station at the time realized the significance and news value of the maneuver. By that evening, the newspapers were

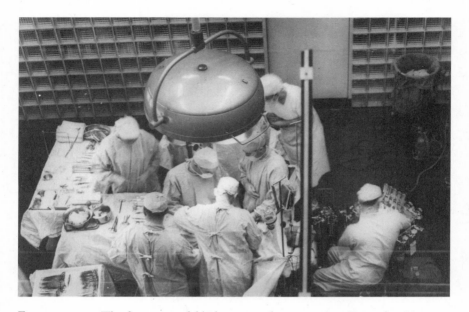

FIGURE 13.1   The first successful kidney transplant operation, December 23, 1954.

trumpeting, "Brigham doctors plan daring operation."[1] From then on, local and national news carried the developing story. Ill-prepared for such publicity, Murray recalled, "it was both an education and a shock to discover how sustained and widespread public interest in organ transplantation was."

Richard Herrick was 24 years old. With rapidly worsening kidney failure, he had arrived at the hospital delirious and convulsing. Treatment on the new dialysis machine stabilized him transiently and provided time for the physicians to organize themselves and formulate a plan. Murray was aware that there was precedence for such a step, as surgeons in the United States and Germany had previously transferred small pieces of skin between three pairs of identical twins. The isografts had healed normally and were microscopically indistinguishable from autografts transferred from one site to another on the same individual. Having already become interested in the subject of skin grafting while in the Army and caught up in the activity in treating renal failure ongoing at the Brigham upon his return, he embraced the possibilities of transplanting healthy kidneys into patients with end-stage renal disease. Beginning work in the Surgical Research Laboratory, he

222

promptly produced a reproduceable model of kidney autografts in dogs, extending Quinby's prior observations that organs transferred to ectopic areas such as the neck or lower abdomen could function normally. His findings also confirmed those of a Danish investigator who had reported that kidney autografts fully supported the canine host, while allografts invariably experienced rejection.[2]

However, these favorable results were unique, as most other research groups had found that such organs excreted water abnormally and concentrated urine inadequately. They blamed the impaired function on a variety of causes that included interruption of lymphatics, denervation, inadequate ureteric drainage, abnormal ambient temperature, and sepsis. In retrospect, the clue to the difficulties experienced may have been that they had directed urine flow to the outside by exteriorizing the end of the ureter through the skin of the animal. Infection ascending to the kidney may have contributed to many of the difficulties described. In contrast, Murray implanted the ureter directly into the bladder, designing a transplant operation which would not adversely influence renal function. By the time Herrick entered the hospital, several dogs had survived normally as long as 2 years on their solitary autografted kidneys. He used the technique in Herrick's operation.

It worked. John Merrill, a young physician on the team, rather dispassionately described the striking transformation of the terminally uremic patient in a paper published a year later. "This report documents the successful transplantation of a human kidney from one identical twin to another. The function of the homograft [he used the wrong term for isograft] remains excellent 12 months after the operative procedure."[3] Things were even different in the post-operative period, with Murray contrasting the immediate and striking superiority of the new organ and the prompt recovery of the patient ("exceeding our highest hopes") to the universal failure that he and others had experienced previously with recipients of genetically disparate cadaver donor kidneys. "In those patients, renal function was always delayed, poor in quality and short in duration. The recipient operation performed on Richard Herrick has been the prototype for human renal transplantation ever since."[4] Herrick married his nurse, fathered two children, and proved that any psychological problems stemming from receiving such a gift from a living donor could easily be overcome.

The success of the transplant between this and subsequent sets of twins triggered the emergence of the new field. Two reasons may have

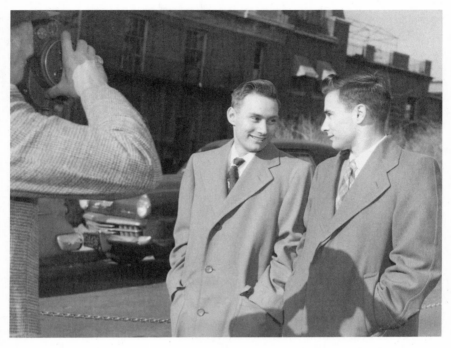

FIGURE 13.2   The first identical twins to be transplanted, Richard and Ronald Herrick, leave the hospital in 1955.

encouraged such a departure from prior practices: the long-standing interest in kidney disease at the Brigham, and the potential availability of dialysis to sustain the patients. The spirit of the place was also important. "The ruling board and administrative structure did not falter in their support of the quixotic objective of treating end-stage renal disease despite a long list of tragic failures that resulted from [the] early efforts."[5] The clinicians who were involved and their department heads, although of vastly differing personalities, worked consistently as a cohesive team over a prolonged period unlike many other larger-than-life pioneers in surgery and medicine who forge new advances in relative isolation and through the force of their personalities. "Those who were there at the time, have credited Dr. George Thorn and Dr. Francis D. Moore with the qualities of leadership, creativity, courage and unselfishness which made the Peter Bent Brigham a unique resource for that moment in history."[6]

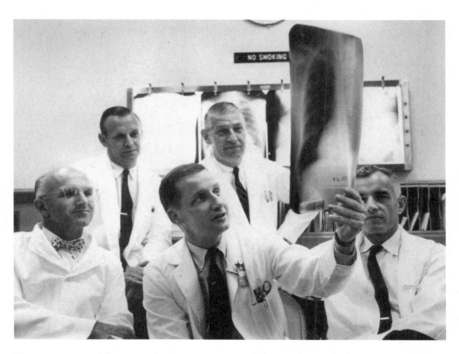

FIGURE 13.3   The transplant team in 1965. (left to right) Joseph Murray, Hartwell Harrison, James Dealy (radiologist), Gustave Dammin, John Merrill.

The "cohesive team" was crucial. Merrill was an original thinker who pushed through many aspects of this radical new treatment perhaps not deemed acceptable by more conservative standards. Harrison was an empathetic and patriarchal figure acutely aware of the responsibility of taking healthy tissue from healthy patients, a startling digression from the age-old tenet of physicians to "do no harm." Murray combined a broad philosophic outlook toward the subject with full knowledge of the nascent biology and innovative applications toward solving specific clinical puzzles. The pathologist, Gustave Dammin, was a quiet and careful scholar whose painstaking examination of both animal and human specimens provided an objective scientific background to the whole enterprise. "As an isolated event, this transplant would have had little significance. The real meaning came from the continuity of effort that had begun earlier with the work of Hufnagel and Hume that had as the ultimate objective the transplantation of kidneys from non-identical donors."[7]

THE STUDY OF RENAL DISEASE had been a subject of interest at the Brigham since its inception. The first two professors of medicine, Henry Christian and Soma Weiss, were authorities on the subject. Weiss's successor, George Thorn, became interested in disorders of the kidney, the adrenal gland, and hypertension early in his career, initially identifying and studying a patient population with "salt losing" nephritis. Then, based on the observations of English investigators that individuals who sustained crush injuries during the London Blitz developed irreversible and fatal renal failure following their removal from the rubble, Thorn began to recognize that some of the injured would recover spontaneously if their water and electrolyte abnormalities could be corrected and controlled.

He also introduced the new steroid, deoxycorticosterone, into clinical use (the pharmaceutical company, *Ciba*, provided him with half

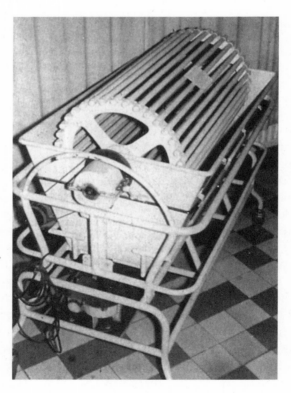

FIGURE 13.4   An early prototype of the hemodialysis machine.

the world's supply), finding that the drug could produce high blood pressure in previously hypotensive individuals with adrenal insufficiency (Addison's disease). By the time he arrived as chief of medicine in 1942, he had noted that corticosteroids could evoke a striking fall in numbers of circulating lymphocytes in the treated patients. Finally, to the consternation of his colleagues, he announced at Grand Rounds that the excision of both kidneys would likely cure hypertension, a startling prospect that stimulated his enthusiasm for their replacement by normal organs; Herrick's rapid improvement after his diseased native kidneys were removed later proved the point. The Brigham was becoming a center for the study of both renal disease and a new class of biological substances, the steroids.

Two events occurring in 1947 solidified these interests and led to a concerted effort to help those with failing kidneys. The first involved three young surgeons faced with a woman who had ceased to excrete urine following a severe infection. There was, by that time, general understanding that renal shutdown developing acutely after a catastrophic event (a massive injury, shock, sepsis) could potentially reverse itself if the individual could survive long enough. Their patient was in this category. In contrast, chronic renal failure secondary to nephritis, unremitting kidney infections, congenital anomalies of the genito-urinary tract, or following inadvertent surgical removal of a solitary kidney was invariably fatal. The conundrum faced by staff surgeon Charles Hufnagel and residents Ernest Landsteiner and David Hume was how to tide the dying woman over the acute episode until her own kidneys recovered.[8]

Challenged by Thorn's suggestion that a healthy kidney from another individual might be used as a temporary bridge, Hume located a Brigham employee who agreed to the use of one of the organs of a newly deceased relative. As the hospital administration would not allow such a radical procedure as a transplant to be performed in an operating theater, the surgeons took their patient to a treatment room immediately adjacent to the ward. There, about midnight, under the light of 60-watt bulbs in two gooseneck lamps, they isolated the artery and vein at her elbow and joined the appropriate donor vessels to them. Upon release of the clamps, the revascularized organ began to function. She improved and the graft was removed. Although her native kidneys recovered completely, she died several months later of hepatitis secondary to a blood transfusion.

The second event related to the new concept of dialysis. During the German occupation of Holland in World War II, a Dutch physician, Willem Kolff, had created a device that could support the lives of individuals in renal failure. This involved the diffusion or "dialysis" of high concentrations of metabolic wastes via a semi-permeable membrane from the blood of those with uremia into an external bath of low ionic concentration. Sausage casing was the only such material available. Kolff wrapped the cellophane casing around frames made from herring barrels, and immersed the unit in fluid-filled tubs. Blood from the subject circulated through the material, transferring its wastes into the surrounding bath.

Hearing about these "artificial kidneys" and intrigued by the possibilities of such devices, Thorn invited Kolff to present his data at the Brigham, soon convincing two young colleagues to work with him to perfect the apparatus. Carl Walter had already contributed substantially to autoclave design and blood banking technology. Merrill had just completed his training in internal medicine and was looking for a specialty. In collaboration with a local engineering group, they redesigned and improved the apparatus. The Brigham-Kolff kidney, now in the Smithsonian Institute, became the prototype for future dialysis machines.

THE POSSIBILITIES OF TRANSPLANTING organs encouraged a handful of investigators in North America and Europe to pursue the subject in the years after the war. But the concept was not new, as occasionally surgeons had previously transferred skin grafts from one part of a patient to a raw surface on another area too large to be closed primarily or with a flap. In the 1920s, Emile Holman at the Brigham grafted skin on several burned children.[9] The healing of the patients' own skin but the destruction of grafts from their mothers provoked him to conjecture about the importance of genetic differences between individuals as well as to note that the tempo and intensity of the destructive process that increased after a second grafting from the initial donor but not from a third party. Despite these and other hints, however, there was an enduring lack of understanding of the differences in behavior between autografts, allografts, and xenografts. Unfortunately, Holman never followed up on his original observations.

Those becoming involved in the subject correlated the deteriorating function of rejecting renal transplants in dogs with changes in allograft morphology and examined the coincident immunological events occurring in the host. These were primarily surgeons interested in translating their experimental findings to patients. And a few took the step. As described, Brigham clinicians had used an isolated kidney as a bridge in an individual with acute renal failure in 1947. Three years later in Chicago, Richard Lawler removed a huge deteriorating poly-cystic kidney from his patient, Ruth Tucker, grafted a cadaver donor kidney to her renal vessels, then joined directly the donor and recipi-ent ureters. The organ appeared to work long enough to allow the remaining native organ to recover and sustain her for five years. Sur-geons in Paris then placed renal allografts in eight immunologically unmodified hosts. All died following the inevitable lymphocytic infil-tration, edema, and cellular destruction of their grafts. Shortly there-after in Boston, Hume transplanted cadaver kidneys into nine recipients. While the majority died of irreversible graft failure within days, he and his colleagues explained the surprising five-and-a-half-month survival of the final patient in their series by the immunosup-pressive effects of uremia as well as by unidentified similarities between donor and host. As dialysis was also slowly becoming a reality during this period, interest in treatment of those with end-stage renal disease was building. In practical terms, however, the universal failure of the transplants muted enthusiasm. "The results from medical teams in France as well as the United States led us to believe that transplant surgery was impossible."[10]

The identical twin experience had shown dramatically that trans-plantation of a normal kidney from a healthy donor could resurrect an individual terminally ill with non-function of the native organs. How-ever, as no genetic differences between donor and recipient were involved, the next step was, as Murray noted, "to broaden the use of renal transplantation in humans beyond that of identical twins. So we, and everybody in the world, were trying to break down the immune barrier. The most apt protocol seemed to be total body irradiation fol-lowed by bone marrow infusion. Chemical immune suppression was just a will o' the wisp at that time."[11]

Occasional clues in the scientific literature suggested that such a venture might be possible. But not until scientists fully appreciated the effects of the atomic bombs on the populations of Hiroshima and Nagasaki did they consider in detail the influence of whole body radi-ation on the host responses. Merrill, a flight surgeon in the Air Force at the time, was particularly cognizant of the consequences. Realizing that sepsis from depression of the bone marrow was the principal cause of later death among those who survived the initial blast, research groups in Holland, England, and the United States initiated studies aimed at controlling or at least tempering the dose. They showed that lead shielding of the leukocyte-rich spleen or a portion of marrow-filled long bone often allowed the radiated animals to recover through repopulation of the protected cells.

Would grafted tissue survive in immunologically altered recipients? Perhaps the most clinically relevant experimental results from that period were reported by John Mannick (eventually to be Moore's successor at the Brigham) and his co-workers.[12] They transplanted bone marrow into a radiated beagle, Sam, then grafted a kidney from the cell donor, Honest John. Sam lived for 73 days, sustained by the first "successful" allograft in a pre-clinical model. This and a few other positive experimental results encouraged researchers working in the field to attempt the strategy in patients.

Responding to the highly publicized successes of the identical twin transplants, increasing numbers of patients with renal failure sought help at the Brigham in the late 1950s. Some brought family members willing to donate; others waited for an organ from a cadaver. Murray remembered that they "had nothing else to look forward to. We could only put patients on the artificial kidney 3 or 4 times at most because we had to cut down on the artery and vein and insert a cannula each time we did it." Emboldened by reports of increased survival of skin grafts in radiated animals, he and his team transplanted 11 patients between April 1958 and March 1962. Each received total body radiation. Several were given bone marrow either from the donor or from several unrelated individuals. The allografts functioned without microscopic signs of rejection, a phenomenon new to the investigators. However, all but one recipient died relatively rapidly of radiation-induced infections despite being kept in a sterile isolation unit (an operating room) following surgery under the most stringent conditions of asepsis. It soon became clear, however, that the source of the responsible organisms was from the individuals themselves and not from the surrounding environment, a finding that emphasized the power and unpredictability of this powerful immunosuppressive modality.

230

The early results were completely discouraging for the house staff, as one of the senior medical residents at the time recounted years later. "Murray and Merrill had attempted non-identical sibling renal transplants on several patients. All had rejected their grafts in a nightmare of dialysis, hemorrhage, uncontrollable hypertension and cardiac failure. The only living result was a disappointed sibling with one remaining kidney. I found the scene depressing, believed that success would never come, and regarded the entire effort as unethical.

"One night, another unfortunate candidate was admitted to my ward for emergency dialysis. The patient was severely uremic and in heart failure. The test skin graft from his donor brother was already turning black. I was sure that if the kidney transplant were carried out the next day, there would be another disastrous failure. My team worked all night to dialyse him and manage his heart failure. By morning he was much improved. Murray and Merrill came to see him and began to plan the transplant. I met with them in the tiny office next to the ward and gave them the final opinion of a man in charge. 'This is simply murder and totally unacceptable. I will not allow this to happen on my ward.' Murray and Merrill looked at me, and each other, with little surprise. They had been criticized throughout the hospital. Few if any members of the house staff or the attendings had any confidence in their efforts. Joe Murray was a calm person who never raised his voice and was at peace with himself. 'That's fine, David. We'll just transfer the patient to the newly opened surgical intensive care unit. We'll take care of him there if you don't choose to do it.'

"I did not encounter the patient again until I saw a picture of him and his brother on the cover of Life magazine. They turned out to be histocompatible and the graft was not rejected. The skin graft had failed for technical reasons. They were the first successful non-identical sibling transplants. The field had begun. Murray's persistence proved to be correct, and I learned that a career in clinical research can be choked with barriers. Only determination can win the battle."[13]

The striking success of this patient contrasted to all the failures and revitalized the thinking of many people about the potential of organ transplantation. John Riteris was 26 years old with end-stage renal failure. His fraternal twin, Andrew, was a willing and understanding donor who was accepted by the team despite what all realized was a small chance of success. The donor and recipient looked different. The rejection of two sequential skin grafts from the patient to his healthy sibling proved the existence of antigenic disparity.[14] However, the kidney functioned immediately after placement into the host, diuresing 32 liters in the first 36 hours. A week later, the shrunken and infected native kidneys were removed emergently. Intermittent small doses of radiation and adjunctive cortisone reversed several rejection episodes over the ensuing months.

Riteris lived a normal life for two decades, never having received any other form of immunosuppression, a term later coined by Moore. As one of the few examples of acquired tolerance in clinical transplantation, this dramatic result broke the "genetic barriers [and] became in principle the single most important case, psychologically and otherwise, in the history of the field of clinical transplantation. The power of the claim was enhanced by the fact that it was confirmed by [the] group in Paris with another fraternal twin case a few months later."[15] Occasionally other successes followed. Thus, by the early 1960s, the favorable outcomes of patients from France, the United States, and the United Kingdom presented an important change from the universal failures reported previously and a dramatic clue that transplantation between non-identical persons could be possible.

DESPITE THE PROHIBITIVE mortality rate from the total body radiation, a few individuals with renal failure were actually supported by their functioning allografts. More successful with the technique than their transatlantic colleagues, the French remained especially enthusiastic.[16] Merrill, who had spent his sabbatical year in Paris examining the effects of radiation on the host responses, was also convinced. But not all agreed. Murray was becoming increasingly certain that an alternative type of immunosuppression was necessary, equivalent in potency but more controllable regarding complications and mortality. X-radiation, he felt, was too complicated and unpredictable. Fortuitously, evidence was arising that chemical agents might provide an answer.

In 1958, two hematologists at Tufts University in Boston, Robert Schwartz and William Dameshek, reported in the first of several important papers that the antibody responses of adult rabbits to bovine serum albumin could be suppressed by an anti-cancer drug, 6-mercaptopurine (6-MP), a state they described as "drug induced immunological tolerance."[17] The two investigators and then others demonstrated that the survival of primary skin allografts could be trebled in treated animals, although the accelerated tempo of a second set response remained unaffected.

Based on these and related observations, a flurry of activity ensued among the handful of surgeons pursuing the subject of organ transplantation. Roy Calne, a young English worker, first reported the results of kidney grafts in canine recipients treated with 6-MP and whose native organs had been removed.[18] While most of the animals died of drug toxicity within two weeks, their allografts remained relatively normal. When the dose was reduced, two dogs survived for 3 and 7 weeks, respectively, before dying of pneumonia. The kidneys showed no signs of rejection compared to untreated controls. Calne had become intrigued with the possibilities of human transplantation as a medical student, an interest greeted with skepticism and discourage-

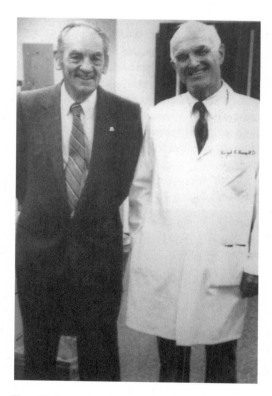

Figure 13.5   Two Nobel prize winners, George Hitchings and Joseph Murray.

233

ment by his teachers in London. Undeterred, he arranged to join Murray in the Surgical Research Laboratory at Harvard in 1960. On the way, he stopped by the Burroughs Wellcome Research Laboratory in Tuckahoe, New York to visit Drs. George Hitchings and Gertrude Elion, both of whom were to win the Nobel Prize in 1988 for their pioneering work on biochemical approaches to chemotherapy. As the two scientists had already synthesized 6-MP, they generously gave the new research fellow several analogs of the agent to test in transplanted dogs.

After confirming the results of his prior experiments with 6-MP, he and Murray then tried the new drugs. A chemical derivative of the material (later known as azathioprine or Imuran) seemed to be the most effective both in regard to its immunosuppressive abilities and its apparently more controllable toxicity. Indeed, a few of the grafted animals survived indefinitely in a completely normal state. Murray recalls this period: "To try to put this breakthrough in perspective, consider our prior experience. For a decade in our laboratory several hundred renal transplants in dogs were performed using varieties of protocols. Our longest survival had been 18 days. Within a few weeks after Calne started to work with us one dog was surviving on a solitary renal allograft for 35 days. This was truly a giant step. By 1961, we had reported dogs surviving over 150 days with normal renal function. It was noteworthy that these animals were not sick or debilitated. They ate well, maintained weight, resisted kennel infection, and even procreated normally."[19] A young investigator working with Hume reported similar findings. It should be noted, however, that in the 1964 summary of his experience with 120 canine kidney recipients treated with 6-MP or azathioprine, Murray reported a mortality of 50% within 20 days after. transplantation and 90% mortality at three months.[20] But even these results had improved from earlier data and were gradually supported by comparable evidence from other laboratories. Optimism, although muted, was increasing.

Conditions in many experimental facilities at that time were by current standards relatively primitive. The Surgical Research Laboratory was no exception. Dogs from the pound were the primary experimental subjects. Anesthesia was usually limited to open-drop ether. Unwieldy surgical instruments made it difficult to perform delicate maneuvers such as anastomosing small vessels. Individual sutures of cotton or silk had to be threaded into the eyes of needles that were sharpened on a stone and used repeatedly. Drugs, particularly antibi-

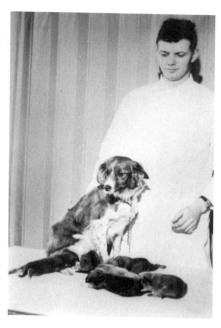

FIGURE 13.6 Mona, an early kidney transplant recipient immunosuppressed with azathioprine. The arrival of a litter of healthy puppies showed that use of the drug would not affect the next generation.

otics, were in short supply. Larger pieces of equipment were often castoffs from the hospital.

One terrifying example of the drawbacks of using worn-out devices occurred in the late 1950s. The standard means of determining the state of a renal transplant was to perform an intravenous pyelogram on the recipient, as dye excreted by a well-functioning organ could be visualized on sequential x-rays. An old x-ray machine was available for these studies. While using it one day, a young staff surgeon working in the laboratory, Nathan Couch, suddenly collapsed, pulseless. He had received an electrical shock from the unit that ran through his body to the floor. The highly experienced surgical technician desperately called the Brigham for help. He and the research fellows opened Couch's chest with the dog instruments and began to massage his heart. Staff surgeons and anesthesiologists raced across the street and carried him to the small ICU. For days he lay in deep coma. Miraculously, however, he gradually revived and went on to a distinguished surgical career. The charred hole in the sole of one of his shoes and a burned patch of linoleum on the laboratory floor attested to the severity of the electrical discharge. The machine still sat in a corner of the room when I arrived a few years later.

Encouraged by the potential for chemical immunosuppression in the dogs compared to whole body radiation, Murray, Merrill, Moore, and Thorn increasingly discussed its clinical possibilities, considering only potential recipients who had no other option for survival. Murray treated the first patient with 6-MP in April 1960. He lived four weeks. The second lived 13 weeks. The first to receive azathioprine survived five weeks. After five more relative failures, however, a critical success occurred. In April 1962, Melvin Doucette, a 24-year-old accountant, received a kidney from a donor who had died during open-heart surgery. The kidneys, cooled by the cardiopulmonary bypass, were transplanted within two hours. Urine flowed immediately.[21] Later rejection episodes were reversed. Pneumonia, presumably resulting from the immunosuppression, resolved. A perforated appendix was removed at 18 months. Following failure of the graft from chronic rejection at 21 months, Doucette received a second successful transplant before dying months later of hepatitis and septicemia.

This important case led to others as most clinical teams turned to chemical regimens with azathioprine as primary treatment. Within 3 years, the Brigham group had transplanted 27 drug treated patients; functioning grafts sustained nine for at least one year. Returning to London, Calne administered azathioprine to his kidney recipients. Hume in Virginia combined whole body radiation, azathioprine and steroids in 6 patients, concluding that "renal homotransplantation is showing signs of coming of age, but is still a highly experimental procedure."[22] The modern era of organ transplantation had begun, as Moore, an enthusiastic and enduring supporter of the enterprise, described in his 1964 book, *Give and Take*.

Late in 1963 about 25 clinicians involved in transplantation and scientists interested in the biology of the subject gathered in a small, hot room in an old building of the National Institutes of Health in Washington, D.C. Thirteen groups from Britain, Europe and the United States presented their total experience with 211 recipients of renal allografts. The results were not propitious: 52% of recipients of transplants from living related donors and 81% of those with organs from unrelated sources had died. Only eight allografts (4%) from cadaver donors functioned over a year. In contrast, 76% of identical twin or irradiated dizygotic twin recipients were still alive.

Only one report relieved the relative gloom.[23] Two young and relatively unknown surgeons from Denver, Thomas Starzl and Thomas Marchioro, presented the results of the 27 renal transplants they had performed over the previous 10 months, most from living donors. They had used azathioprine as primary immunosuppression and had reversed acute rejection episodes in over 90% of the cases with high doses of prednisone. Eighteen patients (67%) remained alive with satisfactory graft function. The genie appeared to be out of the bottle; maintenance immunosuppression with azathioprine and steroids in combination and treatment of rejection with high doses of steroids remained the linchpin of immunosuppressive treatment until the clinical introduction of Cyclosporin A in 1980.

Murray, whose accurate compilation of the data formed the National Kidney Registry, a valuable and enduring resource for those in the field, carefully summarized the results of the Conference. "Although the beginnings of clinical success are apparent, strong reservations must be kept in mind regarding the ultimate fate of these patients. Kidney transplantation is still highly experimental and not yet a therapeutic procedure. Every patient receiving a transplant must be carefully prepared, studied and analyzed to achieve maximum information and to minimize morbidity."[24] He expanded on this theme. "Only the most naive would consider that kidney transplantation is a solved problem and only the most daring would attempt to enter this field without sound laboratory background and the aid of a group of interested clinicians." At the same time, however, he considered the potential of the novel treatment, warning against too Cassandrian a view. "These [survival] figures have been used by some not personally involved with the vagaries of experimental and clinical transplantation biology as a basis for a pessimistic judgment on the entire field."

THE DESIRE TO GRAFT ORGANS other than the kidney arose as a natural extension of the identical twin experience and the occasional successes with allografts. While operations on the liver had traditionally lain outside the existing surgical repertoire, attempts to remove an hepatic lobe or an isolated segment increased after World War II with improving anesthesia and peri-operative support. In 1955, the first report was published of an experimental auxillary graft placed in parallel with the existing organ.[25] Intrigued with the possibilities of transplantation, Moore at the Brigham and Starzl at Northwestern attempted the procedure in dogs, a complex and formidable undertaking. Only a few subjects survived. But with refinements in technique, experimental success slowly increased. In early 1963, Starzl, now in Denver, grafted the first of five human recipients. About the same time, Moore transplanted four patients and surgeons in Paris attempted one. Calne began his series shortly thereafter. All died within days. While several of the livers looked normal at post-mortem examination, those involved called a transient halt to further clinical attempts until safer and more dependable operative techniques could be developed. While Moore and his Brigham colleagues left the field, Starzl and Calne persisted, ultimately advancing transplantation of the liver to a routine and important treatment for those afflicted with terminal liver disease.

OVERALL GRAFT SURVIVAL improved little throughout the 1970s despite critical advances in transplant biology and reduction in patient mortality. With increasing appreciation of the immunological function of the lymphocyte and its role in rejection, investigators introduced a variety of means to decrease host immunity by attenuating or destroying the cells or their rapidly dividing precursors. As experimental data suggested that elimination of lymphoid tissue in bulk could prolong graft survival, surgeons removed the spleen or thymus gland from recipients before or during transplantation. The ineffectiveness and risk of these invasive procedures in this fragile patient population fortunately curtailed their transient popularity. Based on experimental work from Oxford and clinical data from Stockholm, Murray and I depleted large numbers of circulating lymphocytes from the patients via the thoracic duct, the large lymphatic vessel in the neck.[26] Only the initial results were encouraging.

A more lasting strategy to reduce host responsiveness against the graft involved the administration of antibodies produced in animals against human white blood cells. Based on its effectiveness in experimental models, anti-lymphocyte serum (ALS) and its variations evoked much interest as a potentially effective immunosuppressive adjunct. A Brigham resident was placed in charge of injecting lymphocytes from the patients into a horse acquired for the purpose, then collecting blood to prepare the serum. Pharmaceutical companies joined the effort. This approach gained much notoriety with batch-to-batch variation, unpleasant side effects, a few deaths, and many clinical trials. The majority of investigators ultimately agreed that while the material reduced the number and severity of early acute rejection crises, graft survival was not materially influenced over the long-term. However, the experience provided a broad foundation for the introduction and use of more specific monoclonal antibodies as immunosuppressive adjuncts several decades later.

My earliest appreciation of the potential power of corporate pressures involved a meeting I attended as a resident with senior representatives of a large pharmaceutical company that manufactured ALS. Murray, Merrill, and others in the Brigham transplant effort were there. One of our patients had recently died in anaphylactic shock after receiving a dose of the material. Many developed serum sickness. Most had swelling and pain at the injection sites. And the rate of graft rejection had not appeared to diminish. Reasonably, the clinical team had cancelled further use of the agent. The representatives, lofty figures in their organization, were incensed and accused the clinical group of trying to destroy the entire company! They held their ground and the trial ceased. I learned a great deal in a few minutes.

Other approaches proved of more lasting benefit. Tissue matching between donor and recipient became a huge effort in many centers worldwide. The prognostic significance of pre-sensitization of the host by serum antibodies directed against the donor was established. Organ perfusion and storage came into common use. Murray and a committee from Harvard Medical School laid down guidelines about the concept of brain death.[27] With these accepted and in place, the use of organs from brain dead, heart-beating cadavers for transplantation became the foundation of the growing field.

The most significant hazard of transplantation to the graft recipients, however, continued to be the serious side effects of the immunosuppressive agents. Indeed, when I first became involved in transplantation in the mid-1960s, as many as 25% of our patients died in the first months after surgery, often from the sequellae of the drugs. Infections, not infrequently from rare bacteria, fungi, and hitherto unknown viruses, occurred most commonly. Wounds did not heal. The faces of the recipients swelled alarmingly. Their skin thinned. Their bones fractured. The increased incidence of cancer became an unexpected threat. But as appreciation of these events increased with experience, transplant groups embraced innovative methodology and bettered existing treatments to reduce the dangers. Several changes were made.

The Brigham group was among the first to call attention to the excessive mortality rate and suggest means to ameliorate it.[28] We reduced the incidence of sepsis substantially through judicious use of antibiotics and limiting the dose of steroids to treat rejection. The new radiologic technique of ultrasound became an accurate tool for identifying accumulations of urine, blood, lymph or pus around the kidney. Once recognized, the collections could be promptly drained. When we saw irreversible changes of rejection in biopsies of the transplanted kidney, we discontinued the immunosuppression and quickly removed the graft. These and other aggressive surgical approaches to a variety of

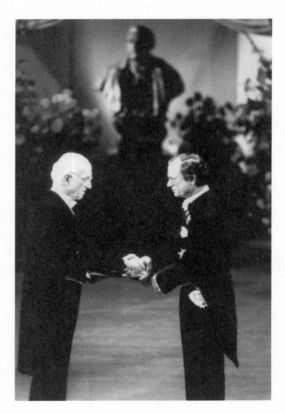

FIGURE 13.7   Murray receiving the Nobel Prize from the King of Sweden, 1990.

serious complications reduced mortality both in the transplant recipients and in the dialysis population. A book, *Surgical Care of the Patient with Renal Failure*, summarized these and other innovations.[29]

The spectrum of achievements in organ transplantation during the 1960s ranged between substantial gains in clinical and scientific knowledge and instances of medical adventurism. The 1970s were generally a time of retrenchment and consolidation, when improvements in care reduced patient mortality and a variety of strategies were introduced to improve graft survival. In this relatively stable period, laboratory investigations shifted from definition of principles to the unraveling of details of host responsiveness initiated against foreign tissue. Several of those who had opened the field directed their energies into new areas. Murray returned full time to plastic surgery, where he became a major innovator in the new area of cranio-facial repair of children and adults with severe disfigurements. His receipt of the Nobel Prize in 1990 recognized his critical influence in introducing a new treatment for human disease. Those of us in the next generation of transplant clinicians and scientists continued to involve ourselves in applied transplant research and improvements in patient care.

CHAPTER 14

THE MERGER AND BEYOND

Much of the success of the Peter Bent Brigham Hospital in innovative study and treatment of disease can be attributed to its small size and relatively few faculty and house-staff. Its long, horizontal corridors allowed easy interaction between colleagues in different disciplines. Members of the faculty, residents, and students lunched together, during which they discussed pertinent topics, interesting clinical conundrums, and potential research collaborations. Ideas flourished, novel (sometimes outrageous) concepts were proffered, projects designed, and teams assembled. Pressures from ever-more-demanding third-party payers, the exigencies of human subject committees, or the murmurations of business-oriented administrators were undreamed of challenges for the future. Even its consistently limited physical facilities and invariably stretched finances did not appear to hamper its activities. All were caught up in the spirit of the place.

The evolution of clinical medicine during the life of the institution, its practice, expectations, relevant biologies, and the experience of those in training, reflected in microcosm changes in the structure of health care delivery and education ongoing in many comparable academic institutions in the United States. In the early decades of the twentieth century, young doctors learned their profession through apprenticeships with private practitioners within the community or under individuals who voluntarily staffed medical schools and teaching hospitals on a part-time basis; general acceptance of the new departures that Halsted and his full-time, university-based associates had initiated in their highly structured residency program at Johns Hopkins developed slowly. Faculty members, often of independent means, received modest salaries. Although they described particular disease states, followed their natural history by examining the patient sequentially, and correlated physical signs with pathologic abnormalities, treatment options were few. Autopsies removed lingering diagnostic doubts.[1]

243

In contrast to physicians who often could do little for the ill except monitor, comfort, and occasionally assuage symptoms during those years, surgeons were able to relieve a variety of physical problems. Examples abound. At the Brigham, for instance, Homans, Cheever, and their colleagues operated effectively on a variety of abnormalities of the abdominal viscera or the lower extremities. In addition to his expertise in a spectrum of neurosurgical disease, Cushing observed that some pituitary tumors produced diverse endocrine dysfunction and that removal of the gland reversed the systemic effects. But in the absence of intravenous fluid replacement, inadequate blood transfusions, and rudimentary postoperative care, operative interventions remained limited. As the century progressed, however, regulation or correction of physiologic abnormalities grew more common. Cutler's opening of a stenotic mitral valve and Gross's correction of a patent ductus arteriosus fell into this category. Accurate laboratory determinations were becoming available: electrolytes were measured, levels of blood glucose quantified, and liver function assessed. The new sulfa drugs began to influence the rate and course of infections.

The period between the end of World War II and the 1980s was generally considered the "golden age" of medicine, years during which "the greatest number of changes in both biomedical sciences and clinical medicine have ever taken place."[2] The outpouring of federal and private money during the 1950s and thereafter encouraged the pursuit of science, while the establishment of the Medicare and Medicaid programs in the 1960s provided health care to the elderly and poor. These powerful societal forces provoked enthusiastic and well-qualified applicants to flock to academic clinical programs and their associated research laboratories. "Careers in medicine were viewed as intellectually stimulating, socially fulfilling, and also lucrative. Despite the length and rigors of surgical residencies, there were always more applicants than available positions." Increasingly, the trainees entered developing specialties that concentrated on distinct conditions or clusters of related disorders. Numbers of generalists declined.

Those in internal medicine and other non-surgical specialties took advantage of the growing understanding and options in treating disease, while research workers benefited from public interest and support of emerging concepts and novel technologies. Many advances occurred. The incidence of infectious disease decreased with improved public health measures and the introduction of antibiotics. New vaccines prevented many childhood diseases. Pharmacologic agents broadened in scope and effectiveness. Novel radiologic methods enhanced the possibilities of accurate diagnosis and therapy. Knowledge of fluid and electrolyte dynamics, correction of acid-base abnormalities, and the development of parenteral nutrition improved patient care. Clinical trials of chemotherapy against cancer were instituted and the influence of hormones on tumor growth assessed.

The spectrum of surgery broadened in parallel. Experience with casualties during the war influenced subsequent approaches to the civilian injured, the burned, and those undergoing complex operations. Physiological changes that developed with trauma and throughout convalescence were clarified. With improved blood banking and transfusion technology, increasing variety of anesthetic agents, and more organized peri-operative care, surgeons became bolder. They carried out radical operations for cancer. They replaced joints, reconstructed aneurysms and bypassed occluded blood vessels. In collaboration with colleagues in other disciplines, they advanced treatment of the abnormal heart by determining myocardial and valvular function in health and disease, investigated new methods of cardiac catheterization and cardiopulmonary bypass, and devised operations to revascularize the ischemic myocardium. Transplantation began to rescue moribund patients with failure of various organs and provide background for a revolution in immunology, biochemistry, genetics, and pharmacology. Clinical studies and research endeavors poured forth from a legion of hospitals and laboratories. Like many of their peers throughout the United States who took advantage of increasing knowledge and technical opportunities of the times, those in the Brigham department of surgery flourished. It was an exciting time for Moore, his successor John Mannick, and their faculties.

BUT DESPITE ITS RECORD of patient care, teaching, and research, the 280-bed hospital, as it had become, faced continuing and debilitating fiscal challenges. The Chairman of the Brigham Board of Trustees, Roger Cutler (Elliott's brother), stressed the problem in strikingly current tones in a major address to the American Medical Association in 1955. "The university hospitals in which medical students receive their clinical training house a matchless spirit of research, and their valuable facilities must be preserved to work for the generations to come. The fact is that our voluntarily supported hospitals are caught in the Big

Squeeze. They are caught in that shrinking space between the upper millstone of collectible charges to patients and the nether millstone of skyrocketing operating costs."[3]

Appreciating the "shrinking space" all too well, Moore and other members of the faculty and administration began to consider the possibilities of merging various Longwood area institutions to increase efficiency, reduce duplication of services, and save expenses. Several were approached and accepted. The Robert Breck Brigham, founded in 1915 by Peter Bent Brigham's nephew, had become pre-eminent in rheumatology and in treating patients with joint disease. The Boston Lying-In Hospital had been established in 1865 to deliver obstetrical and neonatal care. One hundred years later it joined the Free Hospital for Women, an institution that provided gynecological services to needy individuals in the neighborhood and gained an important reputation in reproductive physiology and endocrinology. Their affiliation became the Boston Hospital for Women. Initially interested, Children's Hospital ultimately withdrew from the scheme.

While the very concept seemed grandiose, it reflected a growing trend in the country toward providing efficient, economic, and broadly based medical service to the public. But to merge such organizations, each with its own history, traditions, and culture, took years and often produced sharp and prolonged dialogue among the staffs, university officials, those in city government, and state functionaries. Community activists in Boston vocally opposed the plan to construct a large new hospital and adjacent power plant that would rise high above the surrounding neighborhood. Initial discussions between chiefs of departments, trustees, lawyers, and business leaders began in 1958. In 1971, an agreement was signed. In 1980, the Brigham and Women's Hospital (BWH) opened as a major academic center, the culmination of nearly a century-old effort to create a major teaching arm of the Harvard Medical School. The protracted plans of Moore and his colleagues had finally come to fruition.

Moore retired in 1976 to take the position of book review editor of the *New England Journal of Medicine*. John Mannick became surgeon-in-chief, continuing in that position until 1994 and presiding over the final years of the Peter Bent Brigham and the birth and maturation of the BWH. A product of Harvard and its medical school, Mannick had carried out significant research in transplantation during his residency at the MGH. He then joined Hume in Virginia before becoming chair-

246

man of surgery at Boston University. Focusing his clinical efforts on vascular surgery, he became an established leader in the repair and reconstruction of the arterial tree. Consistently productive as a scientist throughout his career, he concentrated his investigative talents primarily upon the immunological and inflammatory changes that occur in the host following injury.

The new professor strengthened Moore's existing faculty by melding it with his own appointees in a variety of specialties and orchestrating a major increase in the size and breadth of his department commensurate with the needs of the newly merged institutions. In the traditions of his predecessors, his dedication to academic pursuits encouraged and complemented the efforts of surgical-scientists on the staff who were well-funded with federal monies. Many of the residents benefited from this emphasis, spending time in the laboratories and often attaining strong university positions upon completion of their training. This was an especially productive period for the department and its often intertwining clinical and investigative roles.

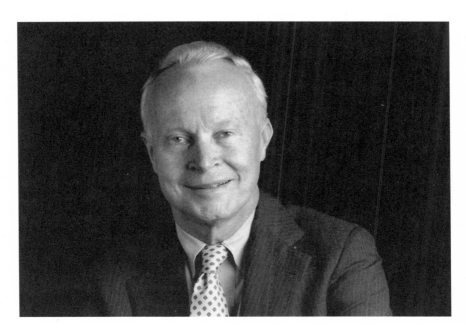

Figure 14.1   John Mannick.

Several individuals remained particularly productive both in their clinical work and their applied research during and following the transition to the new hospital. John Collins succeeded Harken as chief of thoracic and cardiovascular surgery. Interested in operative techniques and refinements, medical devices, and the computer monitoring of ill post-operative patients, he contributed substantially to the growing success of open heart surgery, the efficacy and safety of cardio-pulmonary bypass, and improvements in Harken's intra-aortic counterpulsation balloon pump prototype to assist the acutely failing heart.[4] Realizing early the need for myocardial revascularization, he performed his first coronary artery bypass in 1968, a technique introduced in Brazil that same year, and investigated the adjunctive use of the internal thoracic artery for the purpose. Lawrence Cohn, an experienced and innovative cardiac surgeon from Stanford, joined him in 1971, contributing expertise in the use of allogeneic and xenogeneic heart valves, heart transplantation, and research in a variety of relevant subjects. Collins and Cohn became powerful forces in their field, building a highly regarded program and training an extensive coterie of outstanding cardiac surgeons.

The general surgeons also pursued wide interests. Douglas Wilmore, as noted, continued his studies on the nutrition of ill surgical patients and initiated a successful clinical nutrition service. Richard Wilson, initially involved in kidney transplantation, specialized increasingly in surgical oncology. His large surgical practice and enthusiasm for teaching and research made him a favorite with the residents. Herbert Hechtman moved with Mannick from Boston University. A busy general surgeon, he was a highly successful investigator of molecular mediators upregulated at sites of inflammation, after ischemia-reperfusion, and with surgical infection. For three decades he examined both the local effects of these inflammatory products in involved areas and their influence on distant sites in the body, particularly the lungs. Upon my return from Britain, I joined Murray on the clinical transplant service, ultimately directing it for years. Our group was the first in North America to test clinically the efficacy of Cyclosporin A, a new immunosuppressive agent. In the Surgical Research Laboratory we studied the biology of acute and chronic rejection, defining the dynamics and relationships of specific T lymphocyte populations, the role of macrophages, and the interactions of cell products and their receptors in rat recipients of heart and kidney transplants.

While the administration promoted the new BWH as a monolithic entity and attempted to bury the past of the three merged hospitals, the professional activities of many individual staff members remained relatively unchanged. The character and limits of smaller departments such as surgery and orthopedics persisted, as the majority of the former group came from the Peter Bent Brigham and the latter from the Robert Breck Brigham. Physicians and nurses dealing with womens' health, obstetrics, and care of the newborn carried out their specialized activities as before in distinct locations within the building. In contrast, large departments such as medicine with its increasing numbers of specialty services, anesthesia with its ubiquitous presence in the operating rooms and delivery suites, and radiology with its purview ranging from advanced imaging technology to refined radiotherapy, integrated their faculties more easily into the whole.

The ongoing clinical and research productivity of the professional staff encouraged unity. As numbers of those concentrating in specific fields and subspecialties expanded, collaborations between departments and laboratories grew. Clinical-scientists took advantage of new laboratory space and unprecedented federal and commercial funding to support broadening research efforts. While ties and memories remained in place despite gradual loss or replacement of the physical structure of the Peter Bent Brigham, the new hospital thrived, becoming a leader in multi-specialty clinical services, replete with investigators in the basic and applied sciences, and an important force in medical education. Its partnership with the MGH in 1994 and their subsequent affiliation with several community hospitals in Massachusetts thereafter provided additional leverage to compete effectively for service contracts with health maintenance organizations, insurance carriers, and manufacturers of goods and equipment. This corporate merger has become a formidable power in both regional and national delivery of health care, a theme repeated in many comparable institutions throughout the United States and Europe.

SINCE THE 1980s, a variety of external forces have altered substantially the role and practice of medical professionals in university-based teaching hospitals; specifically, the traditional "triple threat" image of teaching, research, and patient care has become progressively more difficult to retain. Those in surgery are not excepted. Uncomfortable with the intricacies of the new biologies, stressed financially with educational debt, burdened by paperwork and ever-increasing regulations, always threatened by the possibilities of litigation, and facing declining reimbursements from third-party payers, current academic surgeons must of necessity spend more time in the operating room and less in teaching or in the laboratory. To combat inexorably rising costs, pressures to reduce the length of stay of ever-sicker patients in the hospital are unremitting, with the resultant specter of hurried or incomplete care ever looming. The assimilation of new operative techniques such as laparoscopy, microvascular surgery, and robotics, each with their prolonged learning curves, claim additional time and effort. Complex pharmacologic, chemotherapeutic, and radiologic adjuncts to surgical treatment are increasingly common.

With research monies shifting perceptively toward cellular and molecular biology, genomics, proteonomics, and associated disciplines, new generations of full-time scientists are replacing research-oriented clinicians, filling post-doctoral programs and accruing greater proportions of grant support.[5] As faculty promotion within the medical schools is grounded traditionally on scholarly output over patient-based activities and teaching, current surgeons feel increasingly that they cannot compete in the academic arena. Unrelenting pressures to increase clinical output and develop complex technical skills accentuate this dilemma by precluding the time for scholarly reflection so necessary for innovative minds.[6]

The eventual transition of the small Brigham into its large full-service successor exemplified a watershed in university-based medicine throughout the United States from earlier patterns of more leisurely treatment plans and directly applied investigations involving relatively few patients, to emphasis on specialized, high output, corporate driven, and allegedly more cost-effective health care delivery for "clients" by "providers." As the impetus for the surgeon to perform as many operations as possible to protect the "bottom line" of the institution strengthens, not only does teaching suffer but the question whether traditional surgical research is becoming obsolete as part of the long-established mission of a university-based institution arises. Indeed, opinions in the current health care climate toward the place of the surgeon involving himself in answering clinical questions in laboratory models have varied between skepticism by those who consider such activities to be non-productive in an age of complex biology to the doubts of cost-cutting and profit-oriented medical managers who feel that such efforts do not fit into their budgetary planning.

This mindset, often accepted grudgingly but promoted by necessity by many of the new generation of departmental chairmen, named more for their expertise in the business of medicine than because of their academic achievements, will have a long-term impact on those they train. One current surgical chief summarizes the dynamics such individuals face. "Reductions in reimbursement for clinical services rendered, cutbacks in medical education funding for academic medical centers, rising malpractice costs that have now reached crisis proportions in more than a dozen states, and a national nursing shortage are just some of the blows that have been doled out. Their net effect? Make no mistake about it, the business of medicine is no longer medicine, it is business governed by market forces and escalating competition. Few would disagree that these changes have led to an increase in institutional bureaucracy, complexity, anxiety, stress, and physician disenfranchisement."[7]

Unfortunately, many young surgeons brought up in this atmosphere and deprived of relevant scientific nourishment in their daily activities are forced to become business-oriented technicians, increasingly investing their creative energies in outcomes research, clinical trials orchestrated by pharmaceutical companies, and business and management training—subjects foreign to their traditional roles as teacher and investigator. The recent federal mandate for fewer working hours/week and the all-too-relevant wish for improved "quality of life" are additional considerations for the slowly diminishing number of medical students committing themselves to this demanding profession. These issues are changing the demographics of individuals entering the field, as increasing numbers of women and minorities are replacing the white males of prior generations.

Different treatment dynamics are also evolving; successful innovations of cardiologists, interventional radiologists, radiotherapists, and oncologists are gradually causing a shift in some types of long-standing operative approaches. The increasing use of coronary artery stents and catheter insertion of heart valves are providing alternatives to open heart procedures, the placement of aortic prostheses through vessels in the groin are substituting for open repair of aortic aneuryms, and chemotherapeutic and radiologic means of controlling some cancers are replacing operative interventions. Conversely, the demands of complex diseases may foster new areas of study for the surgical investigator that cannot presently be visualized. Indeed, energetic and imaginative young academic surgeons are continuing to bring their skills and patient-based questions to clinical and basic scientists in other potentially related fields who, in turn, are glad to take advantage of the technical expertise and clinical knowledge offered to form jointly rewarding relationships.

To be fair, the role of the dedicated surgical scholar has never been smooth, as exemplified by the interchanges between Cushing and Edsall and other comparable instances throughout the modern history of the field. Moore raised this issue even in more halcyon years. "The surgical investigator must be a bridge tender, channeling knowledge from biological science to the patient's bedside and back again. He traces his origin from both ends of the bridge. He is thus a bastard, and is called this by everybody. Those at one end of the bridge say he is not a very good scientist, and those of the other say he does not spend enough time in the operating room."[8]

For continued progress, it seems clear that chairmen and faculties of surgical departments must consistently cultivate and protect those relatively few of their trainees and young colleagues comfortable on both sides of the "bridge" and with talent and desire for sustained research in applied biologies, encouraging this small coterie to involve themselves early in their careers in the biologic sciences and to translate and apply their knowledge toward specific problems posed by the ill. Indeed, such individuals are currently pursuing the genetic engineering of vessels or organs, collaborating in techniques of gene therapy for a variety of diseases, and other pertinent ventures. Ongoing efforts toward the development of artificial hearts, cultured livers, the growth of myocardial patches *ex vivo*, and transplants of pancreatic islets or neurological cells, are showing promise. Future possibilities seem vast.

CUSHING, CUTLER, MOORE, AND MANNICK were carefully chosen as surgeons-in-chief of the Peter Bent Brigham Hospital. They, in turn, supported their respective staff members who were dedicated both to clinical surgery and to the training and mentoring of the residents, research fellows and junior faculty. In addition to shepherding patients through surgery and convalescence, their sustained spirit of inquiry drove them to pursue detailed study of disease states, a compelling desire to improve existing results, and the design of innovative treatment strategies. As a result, new fields emerged: neurosurgery of adults and children, the correction of congenital and acquired heart disease, the physiology and safety of the surgical patient, intensive care, transplantation of organs, and innovations in vascular reconstruction. Their efforts, extending throughout the life of the institution, nourished a department that was an influential participant in many of the advances in surgery and its associated biosciences.

And they were successful. In the year 2000, for example, the surgical staff of the BWH numbered over 100. Its specialty training programs included 90 postdoctoral trainees. Over 20,000 operative procedures were performed. Research funds totaled more than $12 million, three quarters of which was awarded by the National Institutes of Health. But as financial pressures have continued to build and demands and limitations of health care accelerate, modern departments of surgery are having to re-direct some of their traditional aims and emphasis in clinical activities, research, residency training, and student education. As teaching hospitals in the United States arguably face some of the most disruptive challenges during their histories, it should be remembered that each era has created its own problems and limitations which those involved have transcended and solved.

Although dwarfed and reduced by the administrative and clinical structures of the BWH, the Peter Bent Brigham still stands across Shattuck Street from the Harvard Medical School. Its pillared façade and red brick buildings continue to evoke its significant contributions to the evolution of twentieth-century surgery.

References

Chapter 1

1. Cushing H, Report of the Surgeon-in-Chief, *1ˢᵗ Annual Report of the Peter Bent Brigham Hospital for the Year 1913* (Cambridge: The University Press, 1914), 50.
2. McCord D, *The Fabrick of Man: Fifty Years of the Peter Bent Brigham* (Portland, Maine: Anthoensen Press, 1963), 40.
3. Ludmerer KM, *Time to Heal: American Medical Education from the Turn of the Century to the Era of Managed Care* (Oxford: Oxford University Press, 1999), 19.
4. Shattuck FC, The dramatic story of the new Harvard Medical School, *Boston Med and Surg J* 192, 193:1059.
5. Beecher HK, Altschule MD, *Medicine at Harvard: The First 300 Years* (Hanover: The University Press of New England, 1977), 87.
6. McCord D, *The Fabric of Man: Fifty Years of the Peter Bent Brigham*, 7.
7. Nercessian NN, Built to last, *Harvard Medical Alumni Bulletin*, Winter 2002, 47.
8. McCord D, *The Fabrick of Man: Fifty Years of the Peter Bent Brigham*, 20.
9. Ludmerer KM, *Time to Heal: American Medical Education from the Turn of the Century to the Era of Managed Care*, 18.
10. McCord D, *The Fabrick of Man: Fifty Years of the Peter Bent Brigham*, 128.
11. Brigham, WI Tyler, *The History of the Brigham Family; A Record of Several Thousand Descendants of Thomas Brigham the Emigrant, 1603–1653* (New York: the Grafton Press, 1907), 128.
12. Beecher HK, Altschule MD, *Medicine at Harvard: The First 300 Years*, 320.
13. Letter from W. Councilman to H. Cushing, March 7, 1907, cited in Fulton JF, *Harvey Cushing: A Biography* (Springfield: Charles C. Thomas, 1946), 335.
14. Cited in Fulton JF, *Harvey Cushing: A Biography*, 339.
15. Letter from J.W. Warren to H. Cushing, April 24, 1911, cited in Fulton JF, *Harvey Cushing: A Biography*, 319.
16. Letter from J.C. Mumford to H. Cushing, 17 March 1907, cited in Fulton JF, *Harvey Cushing: A Biography*, 337.
17. Letter from H. M. Hurd to F. B. Harrington, Nov. 6, 1911.
18. Letter from H. M. Hurd to President A. Lawrence Lowell, April 13, 1910.
19. Letter from F. B. Harrington to H. Cushing, Feb. 12, 1910.

20. Aub JC, Hapgood RK, *Pioneer in Modern Medicine: David Linn Edsall of Harvard* (Boston: Harvard Alumni Association, 1907), 308.
21. Letter from H. B. Howard to F. B. Harrington, March 1, 1910.
22. McCord D, *The Fabrick of Man: Fifty Years of the Peter Bent Brigham*, 55.
23. Walter CW, Finding a better way, *JAMA* 1990, 263:1676.
24. Moore FD, The Brigham in Emile Holman's Day, *Am J Surg* 1955, 80:1094.
25. Thomson EH, *Harvey Cushing: Surgeon, Author, Artist* (New York: Neale Watson Academic Publications, Inc., 1981), 74.
26. Walter CW, Finding a better way, *JAMA* 1990, 263:1678.
27. Cushing H, Report of the Surgeon-in Chief, *6ᵗʰ Annual Report for the Year 1919*, 54.

CHAPTER 2

1. Moore FD, Harvey Cushing: General surgeon, biologist, professor, *J Neurosurg* 1969, 31:262.
2. Hecksher AI, *These are the Days, 1935–1936*, cited in Fulton JF, *Harvey Cushing—A Biography* (Springfield: Charles C. Thomas, 1946), 52.
3. Fulton JF, *Harvy Cushing—A Biography*, 59.
4. Fulton JF, *Harvey Cushing—A Biography*, 41.
5. Moore FD, The Universities in Cushing's Life. First encounters: The early years at Yale, Harvard and Johns Hopkins (1881–1912), in Black P. McL, Moore MR, Rossich E (eds.), *Harvey Cushing at the Brigham* (Park Ridge, Illinois, Am Assoc Neurological Surg 1993), 43.
6. Fulton JF, *Harvey Cushing—A Biography*, 68.
7. Letter from H. Cushing to F.A. Washburn, Feb. 10, 1920. In *Anesthesia Charts of 1895 with Explanatory Notes* (Boston: Treadwell Library, Massachusetts General Hospital, 1895).
8. Fulton JF, *Harvey Cushing—A Biography*, 214.
9. Cushing H, Haematomyelia from gunshot wounds of the spine, *Am J Med Sci* 1898, 115:654.
10. Crowe SJ, *Halsted of Johns Hopkins: The Man and his Men* (Springfield: Charles C. Thomas, Publisher, 1957), 45.
11. Rutkow IM, The unpublished letters of William Halsted and Harvey Cushing, *SG&O*, 1988, 166:370.
12. Crowe SJ, *Halsted of Johns Hopkins: The Man and his Men*, 66.
13. Fulton JF, *Harvey Cushing—A Biography*, 107
14. Cutler EC, Harvey (Williams) Cushing, *Science* 1939, 90:465.
15. Cushing H, Cocaine anesthesia in the treatment of certain cases of hernia and in operations for thyroid tumor, *Johns Hopkins Hosp Bull* 1889, 9:192.
16. Cushing H, A comparative study of some members of a pathogenic group of bacilli of the hog cholera or bacenteridies (Gartner) type, intermediate between the typhoid and colon groups, *Johns Hopkins Hosp Bull* 1900, 11:156.

17. Cushing H, A method of total extirpation of the gasserian ganglion for trigeminal neuralgia, *JAMA*, 1900, 34:1035.
18. Towpik E, Tilney NL, Harvey Cushing and his books, *SG&O* 1989, 169:366.
19. Cushing H, The doctor and his books, *Am J Surg* 1928, 4:100.
20. Fulton JF, *Harvey Cushing—A Bioigraphy*, 163.
21. Cushing H, *Intracranial Tumors* (Springfield: Charles C. Thomas, Publisher, 1932), 2.
22. Fulton JF, *Harvey Cushing—A Biography*, 108.
23. Fulton JF, *Harvey Cushing—A Biography*, 205.
24. Cushing H, Realignments in greater medicine: Their effect upon surgery and the influence of surgery upon them. *Brit Med J* 1913, 2:290.
25. Cushing H, Concerning a definite regulatory mechanism of the vasomotor centre which controls blood pressure during cerebral compressor, *Bull John Hopkins Hosp* 1901, 12:290.
26. Cushing H, Concerning the poisonous effect of pure sodium chloride solutions upon the nerve-muscle preparation, *Am J Physiol* 1901, 6:77.
27. Leyton ASF, Sherrington CS, Observations on the excitable cortex of the chimpanzee, orangutan and gorilla, *Quart J Exp Physiol* 1917, 11:135.
28. Wangensteen OH, In and out of the academic arena, *SG&O* 1979, 149:408.
29. French RD, *Antivivisection and Medical Science in Victorian Society* (Princeton: Princeton University Press, 1975).
30. Letter from W.S. Halsted to W. Welch, 1922, cited in Crowe SJ, *Halsted of Johns Hopkins*, 68.
31. Warren JC, *Harvard Medical School Department of Surgery Bulletin*, 1903.
32. Letter from H. Cushing to J. McLean, Jan. 24, 1920, cited in Fulton JF, *Harvey Cushing—A Biography*, 217.

CHAPTER 3

1. Cushing H, A method of total extirpation of the gasserian ganglion for trigeminal neuralgia, *JAMA* 1900, 11:156.
2. Cushing H, The surgical aspects of major neuralgia of the trigeminal nerve: A report of twenty cases of operations on the gasserian ganglion, with anatomic and physiologic notes on the consequences of its removal, *JAMA* 1905, 44:773, 880, 920, 1002.
3. Cited in Crowe SJ, *Halsted of Johns Hopkins* (Springfield: Charles C. Thomas, 1957), 74.
4. Thomson EH, *Harvey Cushing: Surgeon, Author, Artist* (New York: Neale Watson Academic Publications Inc., 1981), 262.
5. Cushing H, *The Pituitary Body and its Disorders* (Philadelphia: JB Lippincott Co., 1912).
6. Moore FD, Harvey Cushing: General surgeon, biologist, professor, *J Neurosurg* 1969, 3:262.

7. Cited in Goldwyn RM, Bovie: The man and the machine, *Ann Plastic Surg* 1979, 2:135.
8. Cushing H, Bovie WT, Electro-surgery as an aid to the removal of intracranial tumors, *SG&O* 1928, 47:751.
9. Light RU, The contributions of Harvey Cushing to the techniques of neurosurgery, *Surg Neurol* 1991, 55:69.
10. Walter CW, Kundsin RB, Harding AL, Page CK, The infector on the surgical team. *Clinical Neurosurgery* 1996, 14:361.
11. Moore FD, cited in McCord D, *The Fabrick of Man—50 Years at the Peter Bent Brigham* (Portland, Maine: Anthoensen Press, 1963), 124.
12. Cushing H, Recent observations on tumors of the brain and their surgical treatment, *Lancet* 1910, 1:90.
13. Fulton JF, *Harvey Cushing: A Biography*, 539.
14. Light RU, Remembering Harvey Cushing: The closing years, *Surg Neurol* 1992, 37:147.
15. Homans J, Harvey Cushing (1869–1939), *Year Book of the American Philosophical Society* 1939, 436
16. Letter from S.O. Hoerr to N.L. Tilney, Nov. 12, 1981.
17. Cited in Fulton JF, *Harvey Cushing, A Biography*, 377.
18. McCord D, *The Fabrick of Man*, 43.
19. Cushing H, Report of the Surgeon-in-Chief, *11th Annual Report for the year 1924* (Cambridge: The University Press, 1924), 49.
20. McCord D, *The Fabrick of Man*, 4.
21. Cited in Holman E, Experimental studies in arteriovenous fistulas I. Blood volume variations. *Arch Surg* 1924, ix: 822.
22. Holman E, Experimental studies on arteriovenous fistulas. *Arch Surg* 1924, ix: 837 and 856.
23. Holman E, Arteriovenous aneurism. Clinical evidence correlating the size of fistula with changes in the heart and proximal vessels. *Ann Surg* 1924, lxxx: 801.
24. Davis L, Harvey Cushing, clinical surgeon, *American College of Surgeons Bulletin*, April 1970.
25. Thompson EH, *Harvey Cushing: Surgeon, Author, Artist*, 265.
26. Aub JC, Hapgood RK, *Pioneer in Modern Medicine, David Edsall of Harvard* (Cambridge: Harvard Univ. Press, 1970), 310.
27. Tilney NL, Harvey Cushing and the Surgical Research Laboratory, *SG&O* 1980, 151:263.
28. Letter from S. Burwell to J.S. Lichty, Feb. 18, 1924.
29. Letter from D.L. Edsall to W.C. Quinby, June 1928.
30. Letter from H. Cushing to D.L. Edsall, March 30, 1923.
31. Tilney NL, Tilney MG, Joint Ventures, *Harvard Medical Alumni Bulletin*, Spring 2004, 50.
32. Letter from H. Cushing to D.L. Edsall, Jan. 9, 1925.

33. Letter from H. Cushing to D.L. Edsall, March 7, 1925.
34. Letter from D.L. Edsall to President Lowell, March 19, 1925.
35. Cushing H, *From a Surgeon's Journal* (Boston: Little, Brown & Co., 1936), 12.
36. Cushing H, *From a Surgeon's Journal*, 503.
37. Cushing H, *From a Surgeon's Journal*, 177.
38. Cushing H, *From a Surgeon's Journal*, 17.
39. Cushing H, *From a Surgeon's Journal*, 501.
40. Cushing H, A study of a series of wounds involving the brain and its enveloping structures, *Br J Surg* 1918, 5:555.
41. Cairns H, Head injuries in war, with especial reference to gunshot wounds, including a report on the late results in some of Harvey Cushing's cases of 1917, *War Med* 1942, 2:772.
42. Cushing H, Neurological surgery and the war, *Boston Med Surg J* 1919, 171:549.
43. Cushing H, *From a Surgeon's Journal* (Boston: Little, Brown, and Co., 1936).
44. Tilney NL, Harvey Cushing and the Oxford Connection, *SG&O* 1982, 155: 89.
45. *The Harvey Cushing Collection of Books and Manuscripts* (New York: Schuman's, 1943).
46. Towpik E, Tilney NL, Harvey Cushing and his books, *SG&O* 1989, 169:366.
47. Fulton JF, *Harvey Cushing: A Biography*, 401.
48. Cushing H, *The Life of Sir William Osler* (Oxford: Oxford University Press, Inc., 1925).

Chapter 4

1. Cheever D, Ladd WE, Moore FD, John Homans, *Harvard University Gazette* 1950, 50:127.
2. Letter from M.H. Richardson to H. Cushing, July 31, 1908, cited in Fulton JF, *Harvey Cushing—A Biography* (Springfield: Charles C. Thomas, 1946), 281.
3. Sosman MC, Newton FC, John Homans 1877–1954, *Harvard Med Alumni Bull* 1935, 29:13.
4. Letter from C. Crane to J.R. Brooks, July 5, 1989, 2.
5. Homans J, *A Textbook of Surgery* (Springfield: Charles C. Thomas, 1931), 1021.
6. Homans J, *A Textbook of Surgery*, 34.
7. Homans J, *A Textbook of Surgery*, 897.
8. Cushing H, Review of Homans J, *A Textbook of Surgery*, NEJM 1931, 203, 1014.
9. Homans J, The etiology and treatment of varicose ulcer of the leg, *SG&O* 1917, 24:300.

10. Matas R, The surgical treatment of elephantiasis and elephantoid states, dependent upon the obstruction of the lymphatic and venous channels. *Am J Trop Dis, Prevent Med* 1913, 1:60.

11. Homans J, Edema of the leg due to local causes, *NEJM* 1937, 209:939.

12. Homans J, Drinker CK, Field ME, Elephantiasis in the clinical implication of the experimental reproduction in animals. *Ann Surg* 1934, 100:812.

13. Homans J, *Circulatory Diseases of the Extremities* (New York: the Macmillan Company, 1939).

14. Frothingham C, David Cheever (1876–1955) *NEJM* (1955), 253:482.

15. Dunphy JE, David Cheever, M.D., *Harvard Med Alumni Bull* 1956, 30:30.

16. Cheever D, Report of the Surgeon-in-Chief, *29th Annual Report for the year 1942*, 61.

17. Letter from C. Crane to J.R. Brooks, July 5, 1989, 5.

18. Cheever D, Anatomy eclipsed, *Ann Surg* 1933, 98:792.

19. Letter from C. Crane to J.R. Brooks, July 5, 1989, 6.

20. Homans J, *A Textbook of Surgery*, 58.

21. Hewitt FW, The past, present, and future of anesthesia, *The Practitioner* 1898, 57:347.

22. Vandam LD, Walter M. Boothby, M.D. The Wellsprings of Anesthesiology. *NEJM* 1967, 276:558.

23. Cushing H, Report of the Surgeon-in-Chief, *1st Annual Report for the Year 1913*, 57.

24. Boothby WM, Present day methods of anesthesia, *J Maine Med Assoc* 1913, 3:1219.

25. Cheever D, Report of the Surgeon-in-Chief, PBBH, *3rd Annual Report for the Year 1916*, 59.

26. Cheever D, Report of the Surgeon-in-Chief, *4th Annual Report for the Year 1917*, 60.

27. Loughlin KR, *A History of Urology at Peter Bent Brigham Hospital and Brigham and Women's Hospital, 1916–1997* (privately printed, 1997).

28. Harrison JH, William Carter Quinby 1877–1952. Memorial Minute, *Harvard University Gazette*, 1959, 59:181

29. Quinby WC, The function of the kidney when deprived of its nerves, *J Expt Med* 1916, 23:525.

30. Quinby WC, The action of diuretics on the denervated kidney, *Am J Physiol* 1916, xlii: 593.

31. Quigley TB, Francis Chandler Newton 1894–1967, *Transact Am Surg Assoc* 1967, LXXXV: 436.

Chapter 5

1. Gordon Taylor G, Elliott Cutler MD, FACS, FRCS. *British Med Journal* 1947, 2: 312.

2. Cutler EC, The education of the surgeon, *NEJM* 1947, 237:466.
3. Cushing H, *From a Surgeon's Journal* (Boston: Little, Brown, and Company, 1936), 17.
4. Cushing H, *From a Surgeon's Journal*, 50.
5. Cutler EC, The education of the surgeon, *NEJM*, 1947, 237:468.
6. Ross FP, Master surgeon, teacher, soldier, and friend: Elliott Carr Cutler, M.D. (1888–1947), *Am J Surg* 1979, 137:428.
7. Cutler EC, *19th Annual Report of the Surgeon-in-Chief, Peter Bent Brigham Hospital, 1932* (Cambridge: The University Press, 1932), 61.
8. Zollinger RM, *Elliott Carr Cutler and the Cloning of Surgeons* (Mt. Kisco: Future Publishing Co., 1988), 19.
9. Cutler EC, Report of the Surgeon-in-Chief, *19th Annual Report for the Year 1932*, 75.
10. Cutler EC, The academic career in surgery. *NEJM* 1930, 102:620.
11. Cutler EC, *Annual Report of the Peter Bent Brigham Hospital, 1932*, 62.
12. Cited in *Harvard Med Alumni Bull*, Summer 2002, 17.
13. Letter from H. Cushing to Henry A. Christian, Nov. 20, 1911, cited in Aub JC, Hapgood RK, *Pioneer in Modern Medicine—David Linn Edsall of Harvard* (Boston: Harvard Medical Alumni Association, 1970), 371.
14. Letter from A.L. Lowell to H. Cushing, Jan. 12, 1932, cited in Fulton JF, *Harvey Cushing—A Biography* (Oxford: Blackwell Scientific Publishing, 1946), 613.
15. Price L, Harvey Cushing, in Forbes EW, Finley JH Jr (eds.), *The Saturday Club* (Boston: Houghton Mifflin, 1958), 183.
16. Cushing H, The basophil adenomas of the pituitary body and their clinical manifestations (pituitary basophilism), *Johns Hopkins Hospital Bull* 1932, 50:137.
17. Letter from I. S. Cutter to H. Cushing, Sept. 18, 1930, cited in Fulton JF, *Harvey Cushing: A Biography*, 620.
18. Shillito J Jr, Cushing the Clinical Surgeon, in Black P McL, Moore MR, Rossitch E, Jr. (eds.), *Harvey Cushing at the Brigham* (Park Ridge: Am Assoc of Neurol Surgeons, 1993), 77.
19. Thompson EH, *Harvey Cushing, Surgeon, Author, Artist* (New York: Neale Watson Academic Publications, Inc., 1981), 291.
20. Towpik E, Tilney NL, Harvey Cushing and his books, *SG&O* 1989, 169:366.
21. Cushing H, The doctor and his books, *Am J Surg* 1928, 4:100.
22. Cutler EC, *Annual Report of the Peter Bent Brigham Hospital, 1932*, 60.
23. Letter from C. Crane to J.R. Brooks, July 5, 1989.
24. Letter from C. Prout to N.L. Tilney, Sept. 18, 2003.
25. Cheever D, *Elliott Carr Cutler (1888–1947): A Memoir*—presented before the Society of Clinical Surgery, 1948.
26. Newton FC, In Memoriam: Elliott Carr Cutler 1888–1947. *Surgery* 1948, 23:863.
27. Cutler EC, Public opinion and animal experimentation. *Surgery* 1940, 8:182.

28. Cutler EC, Zollinger RM, *Atlas of Surgical Operations* (New York: The Macmillan Company, 1939).
29. Letter from F.D. Moore to N.L. Tilney, Jan. 15, 1986.
30. Walter CW, Coach Zollinger. *Am J Surg* 1986, 151:730.
31. Cited in Alexander E, Jr., The Peter Bent Brigham Hospital in the early days of neurosurgical training. In Black P McL, Moore MR, Rossitch E, Jr. (eds.) *Harvey Cushing at the Brigham*, 41.
32. Cutler EC, 25th *Annual Report of the Peter Bent Brigham Hospital 1938*, 78.
33. Walter CW, Coach Zollinger. *Am J Surg* 1976, 151:733.
34. Couch NP, On World War II, battlefield surgery, and three wandering consultants, *Bull Amer College of Surgeons* 1996, 81:20.
35. Gordon Taylor G, Elliott Cutler, M.D., FACS, FRCS. *Brit Med Journal* 1947, 2:314.

CHAPTER 6

1. Cutler EC, Public opinion and animal experimentation. *Surgery* 1940, 8:182.
2. Matson DD, Obituary: Franc Douglas Ingraham, M.D. 1898–1965. *NEJM* 1966, 274:801.
3. Matson DD, Franc Douglas Ingraham (1898–1965). *J Neurosurg* 1966, XXIV:944.
4. Davies JAV, Enders JF, Faxon HH, Gross RE, Parsons L, Sweet WH, Thorn GW, White JC, Matson DD, Franc Douglas Ingraham—Memorial Minute. *Harvard Univ Gazette* 1966, LXI.
5. Ingraham FD, Matson DD, *Neurosurgery in Infancy and Childhood* (Springfield: Charles C. Thomas, 1954).
6. Ross FP, Master surgeon, teacher, soldier, and friend: Elliott Carr Cutler (1888–1947). *Am J Surg* 1979, 137:428.
7. Letter from C. Crane to J.R. Brooks, July 5, 1989, 5.
8. Walter CW, Coach Zollinger. *Am J Surg* 1986, 151:730.
9. Letter from J.E. Dunphy to N.L. Tilney, Jan. 27, 1976.
10. Rosen FS, (book review), Surgenor DM, *Edwin J. Cohn and the Development of Protein Chemistry*, NEJM 2003, 102:620.
11. Letter from C. Crane to J.R. Brooks, July 5, 1989, 7.
12. Moore FD, As we knew him, the Eighth Annual Donald D. Matson Memorial Lecture, 1980.
13. Thorn GW, Forsham PH, Frawley TF, Hill SR Jr., Roche M, Staehalin B, Wilson DL, The clinical usefulness of ACTH and cortisone. *NEJM* 1950, 242:783.
14. Merrill JP, The role of the adrenal in hypertension. *Ann Int Med* 1952, 37:966.

15. Harrison JH, Thorn GW, Crisatiello MS, A study of bilateral total adrenalectomy in hypertension and chronic nephritis: a preliminary report. *J Urol* 1952, 67:405.

16. Mrs. J. H. Harrison, personal communication.

17. Harrison JH, Thomas Bartlett Quigley 1908–1982. *Trans Amer Surg Assoc* 1983, C1:56.

18. Warren R, Deep subcutaneous injection of heparin. *NEJM* 1951, 244:436.

19. Ouchi H, Belko MS, Warren R, Fibrinolysin therapy: Critical thrombolytic dosages and blood levels. *Arch Surg* 1961, 82:88.

20. Warren R (ed.), *Surgery* (Philadelphia: W.B. Saunders, 1962).

21. Long T, Obituaries: Dr. Richard Warren, *Boston Globe*, Sept. 28, 1999.

22. Crane C, personal communication,

23. Crane C, Use of heparin—gelatin—dextrose in venous thrombosis and pulmonary embolism. *NEJM* 1951, 245:926.

24. Crane C, Deep venous thrombosis and pulmonary embolism. *NEJM* 1957, 257:147.

25. Crane C, Femoral vs. caval interruption for venous thromboembolism. *NEJM* 1964, 270:819.

26. Gazzaniga AB, Cahill JL, Replogle RL, Tilney NL, Changes in blood volume and renal function following ligation of the inferior vena cava. *Surg* 1967, 62:417.

27. Cutler EC, Pulmonary embolectomy. *NEJM* 1933, 209:1265.

28. Ochsner A, cited in Steenberg RW, Warren R, Wilson RE, Rudolf LE, A new look at pulmonary embolectomy. *SG&O* 1958, 107:214.

29. Steenberg, RW, Warren R, Wilson RE, Rudolf LE, A new look at pulmonary embolectomy. *SG&O* 1958, 107:214.

Chapter 7

1. Laufman H, Carl Walter's half century of achievement in asepsis. *Am J Surg* 1984, 148:565.

2. Walter CW, Learning from the masters. *Harvard Medical Bulletin*, Spring 1991, 41.

3. Walter CW, Coach Zollinger. *Am J Surg* 1986, 151:730.

4. Walter CW, Finding a better way. *JAMA* 1990, 263:1675.

5. Brooks JR, Carl W. Walter M.D.: Surgeon, investor, industrialist. *Am J Surg* 1984, 148:555.

6. Fulton JW, *Harvey Cushing—A Biography* (Springfield: Charles C. Thomas, 1946), 223.

7. Walter CW. Finding a better way. *JAMA* 1990, 263:1677.

8. Walter CW, personal communication.

9. Walter CW, *Aseptic Treatment of Wounds* (New York: Macmillan, 1948).

10. Homans J, *Textbook of Surgery* (Springfield: Charles C. Thomas, 1946), 60.
11. Walter CW, Finding a better way. *JAMA* 1990, 263:1678.
12. Walter CW, Invention and development of the blood bag. *Vox Sang* 1984, 47:318.
13. Soutter L, Surgenor DM, Reflections of a blood transfusion. *Am J Surg* 1984, 148:562.
14. Cushing H, Report of the Surgeon-in-Chief *15th Annual Report of the Peter Bent Brigham Hospital* (Cambridge: the University Press, 1928), 81.
15. Cutler E, *32nd Annual Report* (1945), 50.
16. Letter from R. Zollinger to N.L. Tilney, February 13, 1976, 1.
17. Dunphy JE, Report on the state of the Surgical Research Laboratory, November 3, 1939.
18. Tilney NL, Carl Walter and the evolution of the Surgical Research Laboratory, 1937–1949. *Am J Surg* 1984, 148:584.
19. Cutler E, *25th Annual Report* (1938), 78.
20. Moore FD, *37th Annual Report* (1950), 38.
21. Letter from J.E. Dunphy to N.L. Tilney, January 27, 1976.
22. Newton FC, *31st Annual Report* (1944), 40.
23. Letter from F.D. Moore to N.L. Tilney, January 15, 1986.
24. Letter from R. Zollinger to N.L. Tilney, February 13, 1976, 3.
25. Moore FD, *35th Annual Report* (1949), 53.

CHAPTER 8

1. Cushing H, Branch JRB, Experimental and clinical notes on chronic valvular lesions in the dog and their possible relation to a future surgery of the cardiac valves. *J Med Res* 1908, 17:471.
2. MacCallum WG, On the teaching of the pathological physiology. *Johns Hopkins Hospital Bulletin* 1906, 17:251.
3. Tilney NL, Cushing, Cutler and the mitral valve. *SG&O* 1981, 152:91.
4. Brunton L, Preliminary note on the possibility of treating mitral stenosis by surgical method. *Lancet* 1902, i:352.
5. Tuffier T, La chirurgie du coeur *15th Cong. International Chir Paris* (1920, 1921), 5.
6. Allen DS, Graham EA, Intracardiac surgery—a new method. *JAMA* 1922, 79:1028.
7. Cutler EC, Levine, SA, Beck CS, The surgical treatment of mitral stenosis. *Arch Surg* 1924, 9:689.
8. Beck CS, Cutler EC, A cardiovalvulotome. *J Expt Med* 1924, 40:375.
9. Cutler EC, Levine SA, Cardiotomy and valvulotomy for mitral stenosis. Experimental observations and clinical notes concerning an operated case with recovery. *Boston Med & Surg J* 1923, 188:1023.

10. Cutler EC, Beck CS, The present status of the surgical procedures on chronic valvular disease of the heart. *Arch Surg* 1928, 18:403.
11. Beck CS, Moore RL, The significance of the pericardium in relation to surgery of the heart. *Arch Surg* 1925, 11:550.
12. Cutler EC, Beck CS, Surgery of the heart and pericardium. *Nelson Loose-Leaf Surgery* (New York: Thos. Nelson & Son, 1924), Chapter IV:233.
13. Jonnesco T, Traitment chirurgical de l'angine de poitrine par la resection du sympathetique cervico thoracique. *Bull de l'Acad de Med* 1920, 84:83.
14. Cannon WB, Lewis JT, Brilton SW, Dispensibility of sympathetic division of autonomic nervous system. *Boston Med Surg J* 1927, 197:514.
15. Levine SA, Cutler EC, Eppinger EC, Thyroidectomy in the treatment of advanced congestive heart failure and angina pectoris. *NEJM* 1933, 209:667.
16. Cutler EC, Schnitlar MT, Total thyroidectomy for angina pectoris. *Ann Surg* 1934, 100:578.
17. Shambaugh P, Cutler EC, Total thyroidectomy in angina pectoris. *Am Heart J* 1934, 19:221.
18. Beck SC, A new blood supply to the heart by operation. *SG&O* 1935, 61:407.
19. Fateux M, Surgical treatment of angina pectoris experiencing with ligation of the great cardiac vein and pericoronary neurectomy. *Ann Surg* 1946, 124:1041.
20. Cutler EC, Summary of experiences up to date in the surgical treatment of angina pectoris. *Am J Med Sci* 1927, 173:613.

CHAPTER 9

1. Zollinger RM, *Elliott Carr Cutler and the Cloning of Surgeons* (Mount Kisko: Futura Publishing Company, 1988), 17.
2. Cutler EC, The Education of the Surgeon, *NEJM* 1947, 237:466.
3. Letter from J.L. Rowbotham to N.L. Tilney, July 7, 2004.
4. Prout C, personal communication.
5. Moore FD, Surgical Professor for three eventful decades. *JAMA* 1990, 264:3185.
6. Moore FD, *A Miracle and a Privilege* (Washington D.C.: Joseph Henry Press, 1995), 54.
7. Moore FD, *A Miracle and a Privilege*, 62.
8. Moore FD, *A Miracle and a Privilege*, 56.
9. Cope O, Moore FD, A study of capillary permeability in experimental burns and burn shock using radioactive dyes in blood and lymph. *J Clin Invest* 1944, 23:241.
10. Moore FD, Sweeney DN, Jr, Cope O, Rawson RW, Means JA, The use of thiouracil in the preparation of patients with hyperthyroidism for thyroidectomy. *Ann Surg* 1944, 120:152.

11. Moore FD, The gastrointestinal tract and the acute abdomen, in Warren R (ed.), *Surgery* (Philadelphia: W.B. Saunders, 1963), 764.

12. Zollinger RM, *Elliott Carr Cutler and the Cloning of Surgeons*, 33.

13. Dragstedt LD, Owens FM, Jr, Supradiaphragmatic sections of vagus nerves in treatment of duodenal ulcer. *Proc Soc Expt Biol. & Med*, 1943, 53:152.

14. Moore FD, Chapman WP, Schultz MD, Jones CM, Transdiaphragmatic resection of the vagus nerves for peptic ulcer. *NEJM* 1943, 234:241.

15. Murray JE, in memoriam—Francis D. Moore (1913–2001), *Harvard Medical School Bulletin*, 2002.

16. Morgan AP, personal communication.

17. Moore FD, *Annual Report of the Peter Bent Brigham Hospital 1951*, 48.

18. Moore FD, *A Miracle and a Privilege*, 130.

19. Moore FD, As we knew him. The Eighth Annual Donald D. Matson Memorial Lecture, 1977. (unpublished)

20. Russell PS, In memoriam—John R. Brooks (1918–2000), *Harvard Medical Alumni Bulletin*, Winter 2002, 60.

21. Brooks JR, Sturgis S, Hill GJ, An evaluation of endocrine tissue homotransplantations in the Millipore chamber with notes on tissue adaptation to the host. *Ann N.Y. Acad Sci* 1960, 87:482.

22. Somers Hayes Sturges, (1904–1991), *Transact Amer Surg Assoc* 1992, CIX:340.

23. Moore FD, *A Miracle and a Privilege*, 145.

24. Vandam LD, Anesthesia, in Warren R, *Surgery*, 279.

25. Garfield J, personal communication.

26. Moore FD, Donald Darrow Matson, 1913–1969, *Harvard Med Alumni Bull*, 1969, 43:78.

27. Matson DD, A new operation for the treatment of communicating hydrocephalus. *J Neurosurg* 1949, 6:238.

28. Moore FD, Donald Darrow Matson, 1913–1969, *Harvard Med Alumni Bull*, 1969, 43:79.

29. Matson DD, Hydrocephalus, in Gellis SS, Kogan BM (eds.), *Current Pediatric Therapy* (Philadelphia: W.B. Saunders, 1968).

30. Barlow CF, Shillito J, Jr, Sweet WH, Tyler HR, Moore FD, Donald Darrow Matson. Faculty of Medicine—Memorial Minute, *Harvard Univ Gazette* 1970, 65:35.

31. Moore FD (personal communcation).

CHAPTER 10

1. Bartlett RH, Surgery, science, and respiratory failure. *J Ped Surg* 1997, 32:401.

2. Cutler EC, *Annual Report of the Surgeon-in-Chief, Peter Bent Brigham Hospital, 1933* (Cambridge: Harvard University Press, 1933), 62.

3. Gross RE, Hubbard JP, Surgical ligation of a patent ductus arteriosis: report of the first successful case. *JAMA* 1939, 112:729.

4. Bartlett RH, Surgery, science, and respiratory failure. *J Ped Surg* 1997, 32:403.

5. Abbott ME, *Atlas of Congenital Diseases* (New York: Am Heart Assoc, 1936), 60.

6. Strieder JW, Attempt to obliterate patent ductus arteriosis in patient with subacute bacterial endocarditis. *Am Heart J* 1938, 15:621.

7. Gross RE, Complete surgical division of the patent ductus arteriosis. A report of 14 successful cases. *SG&O* 1944, 78:36.

8. Gross RE, Hufnagel CA, Coarctation of the aorta. Experimental studies regarding its surgical correction. *NEJM* 1945, 233:287.

9. Gross RE, Surgical correction for coarctation of the aorta. *Surgery* 1945, 18:673.

10. Crafoord C, Nylin G, Congenital coarctation of the aorta and its surgical treatment. *J Thor Surg* 1945, 14:347.

11. Pierce EC, Gross RE, Bill AH, Jr, Merrill K, Jr, Tissue culture evaluation of the viability of blood vessels stored by refrigeration. *Ann Surg* 1949, 129:333.

12. Gross RE, Treatment of certain aortic coarctation by homologous grafts: a report of 19 cases. *Ann Surg* 1951, 134:753.

13. Meeker IA, Jr, Gross RE, Low-temperature sterilization of organic tissue by high-voltage cathode ray irradiation. *Science* 1951, 114:283.

14. Eastcott HG, Hufnagel CA, The preservation of arterial grafts by freezing. *Surgical Forum, American College of Surgeons, 1950* (Philadelphia: W.B. Saunders Co., 1951).

15. Letter from J.L. Rowbotham to N.L. Tilney, June 10, 2004.

16. Voorhees AB, Jr, Jaretzki A, III, Blakemore AH, The use of tubes constructed from Vinyon "N" cloth in bridging arterial defects. *Ann Surg* 1952, 135:332.

17. Hufnagel CA, Permanent intubation of the thoracic aorta. *Arch Surg* 1947, 54:382.

18. Hufnagel CA, The use of rigid and flexible plastic prosthesis for arterial replacement. *Surg* 1955, 37:165.

19. Moore FD, *A Miracle, A Privilege* (Washington, D.C.: Joseph Henry Press, 1995), 228.

20. Moore FD, personal communication.

21. Weed LC, Jacobson C, Cushing H, Further studies on the role of the hypophysis in the metabolism of carbohydrates: The autonomic control of the pituitary gland. *Johns Hopkins Hosp Bull* 1913, 24:40.

22. Moore FD, *Annual Report of the Peter Bent Brigham Hospital* (1956), 86.

23. Hume DM, The role of the hypothalamus in the pituitary—adrenal cortical response to stress. *J Clin Invest* 1949, 28:790.

24. Ganong WF, Fredrickson DS, Hume DM, The effect of hypothalamic lesions on thyroid function in the dog. *Endocrine* 1955, 57:355.

25. Moore FD, *Annual Report of the Peter Bent Brigham Hospital* (1952), 87.

CHAPTER II

1. Moore FD, Report of the Surgeon-in-Chief, *Annual Report of the Peter Bent Brigham Hospital, 1949* (Cambridge: Harvard University Press, 1950), 58.
2. Cutler EC, *Annual Report of the Peter Bent Brigham Hospital, 1946.* 71.
3. Moore FD, *Annual Report of the Peter Bent Brigham Hospital, 1950. 67.*
4. Cope O, Moore FD, A study of capillary permeability in experimental burns and burn shock using radioactive dyes in blood and lymph, *J Clin Invest* 1944, 23:241.
5. Letter from F.D. Moore to N.L. Tilney, January 15, 1986.
6. Moore FD, *A Miracle, A Privilege* (Washington, D.C.: Joseph Henry Press, 1995), 108.
7. Moore FD, The use of isotopes in surgical research, *SG&O* 1998, 86:129.
8. Moore FD, *A Miracle, A Privilege*, 110.
9. Culebras JM, Fitzgerald GF, Brennan MF, et al.. Total body water and the exchangeable hydrogen. II. A review of comparative data from animals based on isotope dilution and desiccation, with a report of new data from the rat. *Am J Physiol* 1977, 232:R60.
10. Moore FD, Surgical nutrition, *Nutrition Reviews* 1948, 6:161.
11. Dudrick SJ, Wilmore DW, Vars HM, Rhoads JE, Long-term total parenteral nutrition with growth, development, and positive nitrogen balance. *Surgery* 1968, 64:134.
12. Moore FD, *A Miracle, A Privilege*, 388.
13. Moore FD, Metabolism in Trauma: The meaning of definitive surgery—The wound, the endocrine gland, and metabolism, *Harvey Lectures*, 52:74, 1956–1957.
14. Moore FD, *Metabolic Care of the Surgical Patient* (Philadelphia: W.B. Saunders, 1959), vii.
15. Brennan M, personal communication.
16. Wilson RE, Jessiman AC, Moore FD, Severe exacerbation of cancer of the breast after oophorectomy and adrenalectomy: report of four cases. *NEJM* 1958, 258:312.
17. Jessiman AC, Moore FD, Carcinoma of the breast: The study and treatment of the patients. *NEJM* 1956, 254:846, 900, 947, 961.
18. Moore FD, Surgical professor for three eventful decades. *JAMA* 1980, 264:3185.
19. Letter from M. Brennan to N.L. Tilney, May 18, 2003.
20. Moore FD, *A Miracle, A Privilege*, 420.
21. McArthur JH, Moore FD, The two cultures and the health care revolution: commerce and professionalism in medical care. *JAMA* 1997, 277:985.
22. *American College of Surgeons and the American Surgical Association 1975 Survey in the United States: A Summary Report of the Study of Surgical Services for the United States* (Baltimore: ACS/ASA, 1975).

23. Brennan M, Francis D. Moore 1913–2001, *Trans Am Surg Assoc* 2003, CXX:30.

CHAPTER 12

1. Harken DE, Foreign bodies on, and in relation to thoracic blood vessels and heart. I. Technique for approaching and removing foreign bodies from the chambers of the heart. *SG&O* 1946, 83:117.
2. Cited in Miller GW, *King of Hearts; The True Story of the Maverick who Pioneered Open Heart Surgery* (New York: Random House, 2000), 4.
3. Letter from H. Soutter to D.E. Harken, cited in Shumacker H, Jr, *The Evolution of Cardiac Surgery* (Bloomington: Indiana University Press, 1992), 40.
4. Cited in Treasure T, Hollman A, The surgery of mitral stenosis 1898–1948: why it took 50 years to establish mitral valvuloplasty. *Ann Roy Coll Surg Eng* 1995, 77:145.
5. Harken DE, Ellis LB, Ware PF, Norman LR. The surgical treatment of mitral stenosis. I Valvuloplasties. *NEJM* 1948, 239:801.
6. Collins JJ, Dwight Harken: The legacy of mitral valvuloplasty. *J Cardiac Surg* 1994, 9:210.
7. Ellis LB, Singh JB, Morales DD, Harken DE. Fifteen to twenty year study of one thousand patients undergoing closed mitral valvuloplasty. *Circulation* 1973, 48:357.
8. Ellis LB, Singh JB, Morales DD, Harken DE, Fifteen to twenty year study of one thousand patients undergoing closed mitral valvuloplasty. *Circulation* 1973, 48:357.
9. Stein PD, Lewis Dexter MD. 1910–1995: *Circulation* 1986, 94:229.
10. Mukhopedhyah M, A biographical sketch of Lewis Dexter. *Texas Heart Inst J* 2001, 28:138.
11. Allison PR, Linder RJ. Bronchoscopic measurement of left cervical pressure. *Circulation* 1953, 7:669.
12. Yu PN, Harken DE, Lovejoy FW, Nye RED, Mahoney EB. Clinical and hemodynamic studies of tricuspid stenosis. *Circulation* 1956, 13:680.
13. Harken DE, Bloc H, Taylor WJ, Throler LB, Soroff HS, Bush V. The surgical correction of calcific aortic stenosis in adults. I. Technique of transaortic valvuloplasty. *Am J Cardiol* 1959, 4:135.
14. Gibbon JH, Jr, Application of a mechanical heart and lung apparatus to cardiac surgery. *Minn Med* 1954, 37:171.
15. Moore FD, *A Miracle, A Privilege.* (Washington, D.C.: Joseph Henry Press, 1995), 224.
16. Harken DE, Taylor WJ, Lefemine AA, Lunzer S, Low HBC, Cohen ML, Jacobey JA. Aortic valve replacement with caged ball valve. *Amer J Cardiol* 1962, 9:292.

17. Harken DE, Soroff HS, Taylor LJ, LeFemine AA, Gupta SK, Lunzer S, Partial or complete prosthesis in aortic insufficiency. *J Thor and Cardiovasc Surg* 1960, 40:744.
18. Starr A, Edwards ML, Mitral replacement; clinical experience with a ball valve prosthesis. *Ann Surg* 1961, 154:726.
19. Collins JJ. Dwight Emary Harken 1910–1993. *Harvard Med Alum Bull*, Spring 1994, 70.
20. Clauss RH, Birtwell WC, Albertal GA, Lunzer S, Taylor WJ, Fosberg AM, Harken DE. Assisted circulation. I. Arterial counter-pulsation. *J Thor Cardiovasc Surg* 1961, 41:447.
21. Letter from D.E. Harken to N.L. Tilney, Aug. 21, 1975.
22. Morgan AP, personal communication.
23. Letter from F.D. Moore to A.P. Morgan, Feb. 23, 1957.
24. Tilney NL, Bailey GL, Morgan AP, Sequential system failure after rupture of abdominal aortic aneurysms. *Ann Surg* 1973, 178:117.
25. Bartlett RH, Artificial organs: Basic science meets critical care. *J Am College Surg* (2003), 186:171.
26. Letter from P.A. Drinker to N.L. Tilney, Jan. 11, 2003.
27. Moore FD, Lyons JH, Pierce ED, Morgan AP, Drinker PA, McArthur JD, Dammin GJ. *Post Traumatic Pulmonary Insufficiency* (Philadelphia: W.B. Saunders Co., 1969).
28. Scannell JG, book review, *Posttraumatic Pulmonary Insufficiency*. *Harvard Med Alumni Bull* 1969, 46:40.
29. Bartlett RH, Gazzaniga AB. Extracorporeal circulation for cardiopulmonary failure. *Curr Prob Surg* 1978; 15.
30. Bartlett RH. Extracorporeal life support for cardiopulmonary failure. *Curr Prob Surg* 1992, 27: 627.
31. Dentighy L, Bramson ML, Osborne JJ, Gerbode F, Hill JD, O'Brien TG, Murray JJ. Extra corporeal oxygenation for acute posttraumatic respiratory failure (Shock Lung Syndrome): use of the Benson membrane lung. *NEJM* 1972, 286:628.
32. Bartlett RH. Presidential Address, *Trans ASAIO* 1985, 31:723.
33. Hanson EL, Drinker PA, Don HF, Van Deventer ST, Bonnet-Egmond J, Veno-arterial bypass with a membrane oxygenator: Successful support in a woman with pulmonary hemorrhage secondary to renal failure. *Surgery* 1974, 75: 557.
34. Bartlett RH, Rolff DW, Custer JR, Younger JG, Hirsch RB. Extracorporeal life support. The University of Michigan experience. *JAMA* 2000, 283:904.
35. Bartlett RH, Dechert RE, Mault J, Ferguson SK, Erlandson EE, Kaiser AM, Measurement of metabolism in multiple organ failure. *Surgery* 1982, 92:771.
36. Bartlett RH, Artificial organs: Basic science meets critical care. *J Am College Surg* (2003) 186:174.

Chapter 13

1. Murray JE, Remembrances of the early days of kidney transplantation. *Transplant Proc* 1981, 13:9.
2. Simonson M, Sorensen F, Homoplastic kidney transplantation in dogs. *Acta Chir Scand* 1949, 99:61.
3. Merrill JP, Murray JE, Harrison JH, Guild WR, Successful homotransplantations of the human kidney between identical twins. *JAMA* 1956, 160:277.
4. Murray JE, Reflections on the first successful kidney transplant. *World J Surg* 1982, 6:372.
5. Moore FD, *Annual Report of the Surgeon-in-Chief, Peter Bent Brigham Hospital, 1955* (Cambridge: The University Press, 1955), 78.
6. Murray JE, Reflections on the first successful kidney transplant. *World J Surg* 1982, 6:374.
7. Starzl TE, The landmark identical twin case. *JAMA* 1984, 251:2572.
8. Moore FD. *Give and Take* (Philadelphia: W.B. Saunders, 1964), 15.
9. Holman E, Protein sensitization in isoskingrafting: Is the latter of practical value. *SG&O* 1924, 38:100.
10. Küss R, Teinturier J, Milliez P, Quelques essais de greffe de rein chez l'homme. *Memoires de l'Académie Chirurgique* 1951, 77:755.
11. Landmarks: Murray JE, Merrill JP, Dammin GJ, Dealy JB, Jr, Walter CW, Brooke MS, Wilson RE, Study on transplantation immunity after total body irradiation in clinical and experimental investigations. *J Nat Inst Health Res* 1993, 5:69.
12. Mannick JA, Lochte HL, Jr, Ashley CA, Thomas ED, Ferrebee JW, A functioning kidney homotransplant in the dog. *Surgery* 1959, 46:821.
13. Nathan DG, Determination can win the battle. *Lancet* 2004, 364:301.
14. Murray JE, Harrison JH, Surgical management of fifty patients including eighteen pairs of twins. *Am J Surg* 1963, 105:205.
15. Starzl TC, The landmark identical twins case. *JAMA* 1984, 251:2574.
16. Hamburger J, Vaysse J, Crosnier J, Tubiana M, Lalanne CM, Antoine B, Auvert J, Soulier J-P, Dormont J, Salmon CH, Maisonnet M, Amiel J-L, Transplantation d'un rein entre jumeaux non-monozygotes aprés irradiation. *Presse Médicale Paris* 1959, 67:1771.
17. Schwartz R, Dameshek W, Drug induced immunological tolerance. *Nature* 1959, 183:1682.
18. Calne RY, Recollection from the laboratory to the clinic. In Teraski PI (ed.), *History of Transplantation: Thirty-five Recollections* (Los Angeles: UCLA Tissue Typing Laboratories, 1991), 227.
19. Murray JE, Remembrances of the early days of kidney transplantation. *Transplant Proc* 1981, 13:10.
20. Murray JE, Sheil AGR, Moseley R, Knight P, McGavic JD, Dammin GJ, Analysis of mechanisms of immunosuppressive drugs in renal homotransplantation. *Ann Surg* 1964, 160:449.

21. Murray JE, Merrill JP, Harrison JH, Wilson RE, Dammin GJ, Prolonged survival of human-kidney homografts by immunosuppressive drug therapy. *NEJM* 1963 268:1315.
22. Hume DM, Magee JH, Kauffman HM, Jr, Rittenbury MS, Prout GR, Jr, Renal homotransplantation in man in modified recipients. *Ann Surg* 1963, 158:608.
23. Starzl TE, Marchioro TL, Waddell WR, The reversal of rejection in human renal homografts with subsequent development of homograft tolerance. *SG&O* 1963, 117:385.
24. Murray JE (ed.), Human Kidney Transplant Conference. *Transplant* 1964, 2:147.
25. Welch CS, A note on transplantation of the whole liver in dogs. *Transplant Bull* 1955, 2:54.
26. Tilney NL, Atkinson JC, Murray JE, The immunosuppressive effect of thoracic duct drainage in human kidney transplantation. *Ann Int Med* 1970, 72:59.
27. Report of the ad hoc committee of the Harvard Medical School to examine a definition of brain death. A definition of irreversible coma. *JAMA* 1968, 205:337.
28. Tilney NL, Strom TB, Vineyard GC, Merrill JP, Factors contributing to the declining mortality rate in renal transplantation. *NEJM* 1978, 299:1321.
29. Tilney NL, Lazarus JM, *Surgical Care of the Patient with Renal Failure* (Philadelphia: W.B. Saunders Co., 1982).

CHAPTER 14

1. Gill GN, The end of the physician-scientist? *American Scholar.* Summer, 1984, 352.
2. Barker CF, Is surgical science dead? *J Am Col Bull* 2004, 198:1.
3. Cutler R, Let's save the goose that lays the golden eggs. *JAMA* 1956, 160:282.
4. Letter from J.H. Sanders, Jr. to N.L. Tilney, Sept. 22, 2003.
5. Nathan DG, Wilson JD, Clinical research and the NIH—a report card, *NEJM* 2003, 349:1860.
6. Zuger A, Dissatisfaction with medical practice. *NEJM* 2004, 350:69.
7. Souba WW, The new leader: New demands in a changing, turbulent environment. *J Am Col Surg* 2003, 197:79.
8. Moore FD, The university in American surgery. *Surgery* 1958, 44:1.

INDEX